PB
617.601   Doundoulakis, James.
DOU
          The perfect smile.

$15.95

DATE			

ile

The Perfect Smile

*The Complete Guide to Cosmetic Dentistry
From Tooth Whitening and Bleaching to
Veneers and Implants*

James H. Doundoulakis, DMD, MS, FACD
and Warren Strugatch

healthyliving**books**

New York

Healthy Living Books
Hatherleigh Press
5-22 46th Avenue, Suite 200
Long Island City, NY 11101
www.healthylivingbooks.com

Library of Congress Cataloging-in-Publication Data
Doundoulakis, James
    The perfect smile / James Doundoulakis, Warren Strugatch.
        p. cm.
    ISBN 1-57826-095-7 (paper : alk. paper)
Dentistry—Aesthetic aspects. 2. Dental care. 3. Teeth—Care and hygiene. I. Strugatch, Warren. II. Title.

RK60.7 .D68 2002
617.6"01—dc21
2002027640

All Hatherleigh Press titles are available for bulk purchase, special promotions, and premiums. For more information, please contact the manager of our Special Sales Department at 1-800-528-2550.

Cover & interior design by Tai Blanche

Printed in Canada
10 9 8 7 6 5 4 3 2 1

Table of Contents

Preface

The Perfect Smile, to me, is not merely a flashy display of white teeth. It is a number of things connected to health and self-esteem. It is as much about what you can do for yourself as it is what I, or any dentist, can do for you in terms of cosmetic dental rehabilitation.

Cosmetic dentistry today is a fast-growing specialty that offers a wide array of new technologies and new procedures that combine to make your teeth and gums as healthful and as aesthetically pleasing as is possible. If you thought that bright, white even teeth are solely the province of Hollywood stars, read on. From this book you'll learn the options in cosmetic dentistry that are now available to you—and how to decide which are best for you.

But the Perfect Smile really begins with you. Ultimately, it is your Perfect Smile that this book concerns. And the responsibility of shaping that Perfect Smile begins with you. It begins when you make that commitment to your own health and well-being to undertake the effort necessary to achieve the Perfect Smile. My hope is that by writing this book, I have helped people realize that their Perfect Smile is not a mere daydream but a reachable and realistic goal.

The book that's now in your hands sets out what those steps are.

Perhaps most importantly, the Perfect Smile is about the way you tell the world who you are and what you're about. The truth is that your grin speaks volumes about you to others before you utter a single word. Just as importantly, it helps shape how you feel about yourself.

If you doubt any of this, consider the flood of "smile" references that thread through art and literature, music and theatre. In love songs and musical comedies. In serious dramas and Hollywood blockbusters. In classical art and pop culture. Over and over we come back to the smile as a touchstone of human existence.

To smile is to experience the human condition in all its diversity and complexity. When Humphrey Bogart plays the jaded nightclub owner Rick in the movie Casablanca, he attempts to come to terms with lost love by famously asking the piano player to "play it again." Sam complies, crooning that a "kiss is just a kiss, a smile is just a smile."

But is it? There are so many different smiles, really. Tom Cruise's could light up Broadway. Jimmy Carter's helped him reach the White House. Julia Roberts' helped her become Hollywood's biggest female box office draw. And Elvis, whose smile delivered more of a mixed message—as much smirk and sneer as smile, but for all that thrilling—just ask anyone who yearns to visit Graceland.

Perhaps western civilization's most famous smile belonged to the Renaissance model who posed for Leonardo da Vinci half a millennium ago for the painting we call the Mona Lisa. It's a beguiling smile, in part because it's a bashful one. Mona smiled with her lips drawn. No teeth show. Why? Some historians speculate she could have used the services of a good periodontist.

Songwriters, like painters, fall back time and again to the smile to convey not only beauty but that elusive quality that makes someone unforgettable. If I could sing, here's where I would break out into song. I'd warble about the "Shadow of Your Smile." I'd remind you tunefully to "Make a Smile Your Umbrella." I'd vocalize my way, chorus and verse, through the Gershwin chestnut, "They Can't Take That Away From Me," raising my voice at the part about how "your smile just beams."

Often, songwriters use the smile to communicate not just the loveliness and desirability of the one smiling, but also that very human blend of wishfulness and determination. That's really the heart of the smile. It suggests that whatever life dishes out, we can prevail. The smile not only reflects the indomitable quality of the human spirit, but actually replenishes it. Smiling helps us survive.

I think that's what Jerry Garcia meant when he sang, with the Grateful Dead: 'There's nothing left to do but smile, smile, smile." Or what John Turner and Geoffrey Parsons, the lyricists who found words for perhaps the most famous song ever written about the smile, sought to convey when they put these words to the melody Charlie Chaplin penned as the soundtrack for Modern Times.

Smile
Smile though your heart is aching
Smile even though it's breaking
When there are clouds in the sky, you'll get by
If you smile through your fear and sorrow
Smile and maybe tomorrow
You'll see the sun come shining through for you

Light up your face with gladness

Hide every trace of sadness
Although a tear may be ever so near
That's the time you must keep on trying

Smile, what's the use of crying?
You'll find that life is still worthwhile
If you just smile.

The Perfect Smile is all of these things: beguiling and beautiful, brassy and bewitching, self-confident and just plain-out sexy. It is my hope that the pages that follow will help guide you to your own Perfect Smile, that place of good health and self-confidence that communicates the best that we are to those that we meet—and to ourselves, when we look in the mirror.

—James H. Doundoulakis, D.M.D., M.S., F.A.C.D.
January, 2004
New York, New York

When Jim Doundoulakis and I met for the first time, in the reception area of his dental practice in New York City, he told me about his idea for a book. He had been musing over the idea for quite a long time, he said, and looking for a writer to collaborate with him. He handed me a thick packet of research he had compiled on the subject, as well as a table of contents. We sat down. He began describing in detail what information he thought the book ought to convey.

"The book will be called *The Perfect Smile*," he said.

He spoke only briefly about clinical issues. He spoke at length, though, about what he called the "psychology of the smile." He talked about how each day well-dressed and well-groomed people come into his office. Some carry gym bags.

They had clearly invested so much time and effort into their physical appearance and general health. Some were visiting his office precisely because they had recently determined to invest in the Perfect Smile of their dreams.

Many of us don't realize that the Perfect Smile is within our reach. People who would not dream of leaving their house with a brown stain on their shirt or blouse go out each day with their teeth stained from years of drinking coffee, tea or soda—or from smoking tobacco. Their teeth are uneven or in some cases missing.

(Dr. Jim, as I came to call him, used the term *edentulous*. I looked it up: it means having no teeth. I realized I'd be looking up quite a few dental terms, not having gone to dental school myself.)

"These people often don't smile," he remarked. "They want to hide their teeth because they're ashamed of them. But a smile is an essential social tool, as well as an aesthetic pleasure. By hiding their smile, they're socially handicapping themselves. They're also going without an important means of nonverbal communication. By not smiling, they seem less friendly. It's hard to overcome that."

I began to realize that our volume was not going to be a tome on physiological issues, nor would it be a book-length guide to how to brush your teeth (although we devote a chapter to just that.) It would be, I realized, a motivational book. You, our reader, would be someone who realizes that you introduce yourself to others by your smile just as much—in fact, more so—than by the words you say. Your smile is the first impression you leave on others.

As I tried to imagine you, our reader, I pictured someone who takes stock of himself, or herself, from time and time and says, in effect: "Hmmm. This part of me is good. That part of me is great! But this part needs some work."

Then you commit yourself to doing the work needed to reach your goal. It doesn't matter if the work is exercise at the gym, acquiring a new wardrobe, or going back to school to master an important skill or technology. What matters is the commitment: determining that you will in fact take the steps necessary to reach your goal. Then, following through on the plan, knowing the effort will produce the desired outcome.

Think, for a moment, of the fellow eager to get physically fit, but who hasn't exercised in ten years. Our friend lives on steak and ice cream, and has one developed muscle, the thumb, used for selecting TV channels on the remote. For such a person, becoming physically fit is a challenge, but it is indeed possible. Doing so, however, will require a major change in attitude as well as a major change in lifestyle. The latter will not be possible without the former.

If our out-of-shape friend goes to a step class, then collapses after five minutes—and never goes back—the effort would be pointless. The right first step, in fact, would be making the personal commitment to changing that sedentary lifestyle. Then, selecting and beginning an exercise regiment that is demanding but at the same time one that can be maintained over time, and gradually increased.

What happens under such a regimen? Your body loses fat and gains muscle tone. Overall physical health improves. You look better. You feel better. Because you see and feel these improvements, you are motivated to maintain the healthier lifestyle.

Improving your oral health is no different. Your dentist can help. But the real determining factor is you. By reading this book, you are taking that crucial first step towards improving the health of your teeth and gums. In so doing you are improving the overall appearance of the lower third of your face. This cannot but dramatically enhance your self-image as well. The benefits won't materialize overnight. But by taking this first step, you are that much closer to achieving your perfect smile.

The book in your hands outlines the steps that are part of the process that results in a first-class smile. Following those steps, of course, is up to you. The fact that you're investing in this book suggests that you've already taken that first step.

You'll be glad you did.

—Warren Strugatch
Hampton Bays, NY
January 2004

DEDICATION

To my dear friends Gus Bubaris, Tassos Georgiades, Mat Wanning, and Cousin Jim Douglas...for always being there for me.

To my beautiful wife Maro, who has brought great elation, happiness, and love into my life and supporting me during life's most challenging moments...and for bringing our daughter Thalia Areti into this world. The joy our little girl has brought us will be eternal.
—James H. Doundoulakis

To my grandfather, Morris Strugatch.
And to my parents, Jack and Sondra Strugatch.
—Warren Strugatch

ACKNOWLEDGMENTS

I sincerely thank Mr. Andrew Flach and the talented staff at Hatherleigh Press for believing in this book, in its vision, and their expertise in putting it all together. Many thanks to Warren Strugatch for his invaluable guidance and ability in the preparation of the manuscript.

Psychology of the Smile

There is reason to believe we are genetically programmed to smile, and to respond to the smiles of others. When you produce a genuine smile, on the most basic level you are signaling, "Don't attack me; welcome me! I'm a friend, not a foe."

No less an authority than Charles Darwin speculated that our hominoid ancestors managed to convey peaceful intent to other members of their species by smiling, thus achieving evolutionary advantage. While our forebears were literally able to smile their way out of trouble, other pre-human primates were not. Our ancestors used smiling to signal non-aggression, avoiding possibly lethal fights. In addition, smiles were used to gain cooperation from others, an essential skill required for hunting large game. And of course, smiling was (and still is) used to attract the most desirable mates, likely due to the fact that healthy gums portend overall good health, increasing the probability of strong offspring.

The smile, used to reflect joy and good will, is one of four primal gestures humans make. (The others express fear, anger, and disgust.) We begin to smile in infancy, sometimes as early as two days old. We do not need someone to teach us. An infant born blind will smile at about the same age as an infant born with sight.

Smiles Serve Many Purposes

When produced properly—by flexing a certain combination of facial muscles—a smile allows us to communicate eloquently and gracefully. We smile to show respect and deference, to demonstrate a desire to cooperate and the intent to please. We smile to take the edge off a harsh comment. We smile to proffer friendship, and also to show love— or lust. We smile to convey fortitude and acceptance of life's disappointments, and we smile to offer support and encouragement. The smile is our fundamental social gesture and an essential tool in social interaction.

To not smile, whether because of inclination or loss of motor skills, is to endure isolation and loneliness. Studies of patients in rehabilitation after a stroke indicate that those who experience partial paralysis in the face are most likely to suffer from depression. Because they cannot smile, they lose the ability to communicate their interest in the world around them. It then becomes a struggle to connect with others on a social or interpersonal level. Others may misinterpret the unchanging cast of their features—the "mask" of paralysis—as indicative of lost interest. Sadly, in many cases visitors stop addressing the patient directly and talk "over" him or her.

Patients who regain at least some of the ability to produce a smile—often after years of excruciating effort relearning how to use the smile muscles—are far less likely to be suicidal than those who do not regain this ability.

We share with other mammals the ability to lift our lips evenly to display teeth and gums. Only the higher primates do this to convey friendliness; other mammals reveal their teeth as a warning. Think of the junkyard dog curling its lip to warn off the potential intruder. The watchdog's snarl—an asymmetrical lifting of the lip—displays the teeth unevenly, with emphasis on the jagged canines. Most potential intruders get the point.

The Duchenne Smile

Much of our understanding of the physiology of the smile is based on work done more than 150 years ago by the French neurologist, Guillaume Duchenne. Duchenne used a battery to apply electric shocks to cadavers, thereby isolating the 100 muscles involved in producing facial gestures—including 10 muscles that produce the 18 facial gestures we categorize as smiles.

Perhaps the major discovery made by Duchenne was the isolation of the *zygomaticus* muscle. This muscle, which connects the corners of the mouth with the cheekbone, is the primary smile muscle. Researchers often describe a genuine smile as a Duchenne smile in honor of his pioneering work.

To feel your own *zygomaticus* muscle, try this exercise. Touch your thumb with the other four fingers of your hand. Put your little finger on the corner of your mouth and the thumb on your cheekbone. Let your fingertips gently touch your cheek. Pronounce the word "eat" in an exaggerated manner, as if for the benefit of a lip-reader. Can you feel the *zygomaticus* muscle flex in your cheek?

It's been observed that a true smile lights up one's face, and there is physiological truth to this. The *zygomaticus* underlies the *orbicularis oculi* muscle surrounding the eye. When you grin, you work both the *zygomaticus* and *orbicularis* muscles. Your eyes appear to twinkle. Your cheekbone becomes slightly more pronounced. The skin around your eyes crinkles a bit, producing what are commonly called laugh lines.

The opposite of the Duchenne smile is the risorius smile, named after the facial muscle that is used to pull the lips back but not up. The risorius smile tends to strike others as false or insincere, though it is not so much false as it is calculated. It's a smile we put on when we feel obliged to smile, but there is no spontaneity to it. We smile because we think we should, not because we *feel* like it.

Raymond McGraime, an expert on body language in Nesconset, New York, says that the risorius smile often produces an unintended effect. "It's a smile that indicates deception," he said. "It also indicates subordination rather than power, since it is the smile furthest removed from showing canines."

Smiling using the "wrong" muscles often provokes undesired reactions, McGraime says. "In my work as a therapist I help kids move better among their peers," he said. "Facial gestures are a part of overall movement and non-verbal communication. So one of the things I do is help kids smile properly. If you're a kid and you have a 'geeky' smile, you get teased an awful lot. It's possible to put a stop to that by learning the right way to smile. You start sending out a different message about yourself."

From Goofy Grins to Lascivious Leers

Comics have long gotten laughs by producing all sorts of geeky (or "wrong") smiles. Perhaps the most famous geeky smile of the past 50 years belonged to Jerry Lewis' classic comedic persona during his Hollywood heyday with Dean Martin. Lewis pushed his lips out and appeared buck-toothed, as if modeling a how-to manual for how not to grin. Many found him hilarious. Of course, the dopey gesture was intentional, and Lewis was well reimbursed for it.

Actors, among others, learn how to work their smiles to develop their characters. They learn that by flexing the *nasalis* muscle they can flare their nostrils and put a crease in the center of the nose—a gesture that turns a smile into a leer. They can flex the *orbicularis oris* to make the mouth more oval, a gesture associated with kissing and sexual excitement.

For most of us, however, the perfect smile is pure Duchenne. The benefits of perfecting the Duchenne smile are compelling.

According to Raymond McGraime, what happens when you allow yourself to smile regularly and genuinely is that you "train" your face to support the smile. Even when not smiling, your face suggests your manner is congenial. Here's how McGraime explains it:

"When you smile using the *zygomaticus* muscle, it pulls the bone behind the eye. This bone is your cheekbone, and in order to accommodate the stress it becomes larger. This is a permanent change. And it's a good change—large cheekbones are considered a sign of beauty in many cultures, including American culture. And we assign positive characteristics to those who strike us as attractive."

You can bring about this change simply by smiling plenty of Duchenne smiles. Continues Mr. McGraime: "What you're doing, each time you smile, is kinesthetically sculpting your face. You're giving yourself great cheekbones to offset your great smile."

Physiological Benefits are Compelling

There are may other benefits associated with smiling. Studies of brain electrical pulse patterns show increased activity in the left prefrontal cortex—the center of positive emotions—when smiling. Substantial evidence suggests smiling triggers chemicals that serve as natural mood elevators. These chemicals make us feel better, and thereby improve our ability to identify solutions to our problems and act on them. In other words, we can make ourselves feel better by smiling.

McGraime believes these studies are valuable. "We've long known that the mind affects the body," he observes. "But the idea that the body affects the mind is a real paradigm shift in physiognomy. What we're learning is that movement is a kind of pharmacopoeia. Movement generates endorphins, which are chemicals that affect the brain's hypothalamus. By smiling, you produce brain chemicals that make you feel better."

The converse is also true. Some people who don't smile often acknowledge feeling depressed much of the time. An important trend in both physical therapy and behavioral counseling is to encourage patients to smile as the first step toward improving their ability to cope with problems. Some therapists use techniques like biofeedback to show patients the somatic benefits of smiling.

It turns out our grandparents gave us good advice when they urged us to smile in the face of trouble. This folk wisdom had been passed down to them and to their own parents and grandparents before them. They were right, even if they didn't know why.

Others Mirror Your Smile

Another reason to smile is that the gesture tends to elicit smiles in return. You can easily demonstrate this for yourself. Go outside and walk a block or two. Consciously keep a smile on your face and make eye contact with each passerby. Watch as one person after another returns your smile.

Now turn around and walk back, this time frowning. Make eye contact as before, and what do you see? Most people will return your frown with similar expressions.

Still, not everyone smiles. We all know someone whose lips seem permanently pursed as if in censure, with lips arched downward in a perpetual frown. Chances are such people are not even aware their mouths have taken on this negative position. It's just that they've made this gesture so often over time that it's become, in effect, their "default" face.

Sylvan Thomas, an emotion researcher, contends that anti-smile gestures reflect a fear of uninhibited emotion; people "edit" their feelings and facial gestures because they feel it's somehow unseemly to look (or feel) delighted.

The frowns, sulks, sneers, and pursed lips of the smile-impaired soon become fixed expressions. For these individuals, producing a smile is truly difficult—they have forgotten how to smile. After many years of not smiling, the person's smile muscles are out of practice. If pressed to smile, such a person will usually produce a kind of grimace. Ironically, the grimace will strike onlookers as even more unpleasant than the characteristic frown, reinforcing the person's belief that there really is no reason to smile anyway.

The Smile in Your Future

There are people who are smile-challenged for another reason: They are ashamed of their teeth and gums. They believe their smile is unattractive. Perhaps their teeth are crooked, or stained from years of drinking beverages like coffee, tea, and cola, or from smoking tobacco. Perhaps some teeth are chipped or missing. Whatever the reason, by keeping their smile imprisoned behind their lips they deprive themselves of the most vital communication tool we have apart from speech itself.

If you're one of those people, the good news is that these problems can be corrected. In the following pages you'll learn all about how you can achieve the perfect smile you've always wanted.

Chapter 1

A Trip to the Dentist

A New Look at an Old Phobia

You need a root canal." Those five words certainly are among the most stressful to hear in the English language. The phrase "root canal" is universally understood to suggest an uncomfortable situation that lasts for some time. You know things will get better, but you also know that the process is going to hurt.

It will come as no surprise that dentists think about root canals quite differently. To the doctor, a root canal is a way to help patients regain good oral health after their teeth have rotted into the nerve tissue. Though most people know that the dentist's goal is to alleviate pain, common expressions like "I need that (whatever *that* is) like I need root canal," reinforce negative expectations.

The term root canal, which literally refers to the therapeutic process of removing diseased tissue, has become a metaphor for agonizing—albeit necessary—physical discomfort. And anticipation of pain or discomfort is the primary reason many individuals develop phobias regarding dental treatment.

Let's try a quick survey. Fill in the missing words in each sentence.

1. When I visit the dentist, I expect the experience will be _____.

2. The last time I visited my dentist, the experience was _____.

3. The most painful experience I ever had in a dentist's office was with Dr. _____.

Here's an interesting phenomenon: Most people use a negative word in the first sentence, a more neutral word in the second, and implicate their childhood dentist in the third.

For sentence one, people typically use negative adjectives like "painful" or "uncomfortable" to describe what they expect when visiting the dentist. Yet when describing their own recent experiences (in sentence two), they tend to use more neutral language, such as "not uncomfortable," "fairly comfortable" or "pretty much pain-free." (If you do describe visits to your current practitioner with pain-associated terms, be sure to read Chapter 2 for tips on how to choose the right dentist for your needs. Your experience should not routinely be unpleasant.)

For dentists, the third question reveals the most about how early memories create perceptual rather than actual discomfort. Many people with dental phobia draw assumptions from their earliest experiences and group all practitioners into the same pain-inducing category. They expect their visit to the dentist to be painful, and this becomes a self-fulfilling prophecy.

The cultural association of dentistry with extreme pain, coupled with exaggerated and selective memories of unpleasant dental experiences can foster a lifelong case of dental phobia. This fear of dentistry keeps more than half of Americans from visiting their dentists regularly.

The most extreme examples of dental phobia are cases dentists never see. People suffer from debilitating discomfort before they phone for an appointment. Some endure tissue and bone degeneration and even tooth loss rather than step into a dentist's office.

Those suffering moderate dental phobia are pretty easy to spot. They hover nervously around the chair for a moment and then edge into it, like an anxious new swimmer crouched over a pool working up the nerve to take the plunge. Once seated, they grasp each armrest until their knuckles turn white. Their jaws may reveal tension. Their eyes open wide, and stay that way until the dental bib comes off.

The least afflicted simply show up for treatment once in a while. Their visits occur less often than good oral health requires. Any dreams they might have of having the perfect smile remain unrealized.

Where do you fit in? Now is a good time to consider the following questions.

Dental Phobia Checklist

Answer the following questions.

1. Have you postponed making an appointment with your dentist in the past six months because of inconvenience? Other priorities? Forgetfulness?

2. When you do go for an appointment, have you been told by a dental professional that your oral health would improve if you scheduled appointments regularly?

3. Over the past six months, have you made decisions about what food to eat based on how you anticipated that food would affect the nerves in your teeth? For example, have you passed on an ice cream dessert or said no to a steaming bowl of hot soup, and not followed up by making a dental appointment within 24 hours?

If you answered yes to one of these questions, you might have some degree of dental phobia. If you answered yes to two or all questions, you likely have dental phobia that is affecting your health and appearance.

When planning this book, we decided it was important to address this issue of dental phobia right at the start. Many people experience some degree of dental phobia, which over time can contribute to the gradual deterioration of their oral health. Some chose to put off scheduling visits until pain becomes unbearable rather than face the dental chair. This process only underscores the original phobia and can condemn them to years of terrible pain and severe, unyielding discomfort—all of it unnecessary and avoidable.

Most cases are not that extreme. The majority of people don't spend a lifetime avoiding the dentist, but merely skirt the dentist's chair as much as possible. They avoid routine appointments and procedures that will improve their overall health and appearance, and only schedule a visit when their teeth ache. Such emergency-only patients are usually vaguely apologetic about their behavior, but not quite ready to make a permanent change. There's always a reason why they haven't come in earlier.

As is the case with all phobias, the fear of dental treatment is based on a highly exaggerated version of reality. Many people can trace their phobia back to a particular experience or series of experiences in a dentist's chair. Often these experiences took place in early childhood, and in their memory the pain is excruciating.

However, the roots of dental phobia rarely lie entirely in the realm of physical pain. There is usually a strong psychological component. The reaction of the dentist, and the other people involved in the experience, often the mother or father, are part of this equation.

Dentists—like carpenters, computer programmers, electricians, and lawyers—are not always experts in applied psychology. Their approach to dealing with frightened and anxious patients is not always adequate. Until fairly recently it was not uncommon for a dentist to deal with a squeamish youngster by disregarding the patient's discomfort, or denying it entirely. Most can remember hearing something along the lines of, "Oh, it doesn't really hurt," or "Be a big boy (or girl) and this will all be over soon." Often an adult voice would scold, "If you only brushed your teeth, we wouldn't be here, and the dentist wouldn't be drilling big holes in your teeth," and "You eat so much candy, it's no wonder."

Although it's easy to dismiss such comments as insensitive and cloddish, many people can recall intense feelings of dread and defeat when faced with similar situations. The combination of physical discomfort and psychological distress can take a real toll on your psyche at such vulnerable points in your development. Those who experienced similar scenarios rarely forget them. Memories of pain and humiliating denial come flooding back with each looming visit.

Research suggests that powerful sensations endure in memory while routine sensations are forgotten. Memory erases the bland and preserves the extreme in exaggerated form, turning yesterday's mild discomfort into a searing memory of great pain. We forget the 10, 20, or 100 visits that passed without incident and remember the one or two sessions when poking, probing, and drilling seemed endless. Memories of pain endure. When we look back, our visits to the dentist always hurt.

Culture also reinforces this phenomenon. It's human nature to tell jokes when a subject is stressful. So many people experience some degree of dental phobia that the dental profession has inevitably become the butt of a whole genre of jokes. Remember the sadistic dentist who tortured Dustin Hoffman in the cult classic *The Marathon Man?*

Complaining about the dentist is also a socially acceptable form of emotional venting and interpersonal bonding. Someone at the office says, "You guys get to go out to lunch, I have to go to the dentist." Naturally, everyone commiserates.

It's also acceptable to complain about dental pain: "Oh, does my tooth hurt"; "I don't know which is worse, the toothache or seeing the dentist"; "So I go in for bridgework again today. I can't wait until he's finally finished." Society tells us that visiting the dentist is going to hurt. Naturally, we cringe in commiseration and learned expectation, even if our own recent experiences are all relatively benign.

No one says, "Just got back from the dentist. Didn't feel a thing."

Confronting Dental Phobia

There are a number of ways to overcome a phobia, but there is only one way to start: acknowledge that you have a phobia, and that you want to eliminate it.

If you postpone scheduling dental checkups because you fear your dentist, try the following visualization. Think back to your most unpleasant experience, but this time, confront it from your current perspective as an adult. In your mind, conjure the office of the dentist you described when you answered the third question on page 2. What did the office look like from the outside? What did the interior look like? How did you get there? Did a parent take you? Do you recall if you traveled by car? Did you walk there with someone? Do you remember any bits of conversation on the way to the office, or afterward?

What was said during the visit? If you said you felt pain, how was it acknowledged? What about the pain itself? Can you remember what the procedure was, which side of the mouth was involved, and how intense the pain felt?

Can you recall visits that passed pleasantly, without discomfort? If you can, try to compare these visits with others where you felt pain. Visualize the dentist finishing the procedure that was painful, and this time, say out loud, "Oh, that really hurt," or any other phrase you would use.

This time, you're in charge, and the dentist is going to pay attention! In your mind's eye, stop the action. Now focus on the image of the dentist on the pain-free visit. Since most dental procedures are virtually painless, this is the more realistic image. Keep it in your mind.

Some people find recreating this long-ago visit brings out feelings of anger about the way the dentist—and, often, the accompanying parent—handled the situation. In this visualization, you're the one in charge, and you can control the outcome.

If you have been avoiding dental appointments because you fear painful procedures, you will be relieved to know that modern dentistry has made significant inroads in reducing pain and

A Word from the Doctor

In my office, we attempt to minimize disagreeable sensory experiences patients remember from long-ago dental visits and replace them with pleasant and calming sights, scents, sounds, textures, and tastes. We believe that taking this holistic approach to improving the entire experience eliminates the sensory "triggers" that stimulate unhappy memories. Scent, in particular, is a powerful memory-generator. (This is a very primary survival mechanism. If you smell a certain scent when experiencing pain, you'll be repulsed every time you smell that scent for the rest of your life.)

With that in mind, we've eliminated the once-common medicinal clove odor that so often triggers anxiety by association. Instead, patients who enter our office receive a pleasant olfactory greeting: the wafting aroma of apple-spice potpourri and various selected botanical scents. Remember those awful

discomfort. Extensive injections and drilling, post-visit sensitivity and post-operative aching are things of the past. People are often genuinely surprised to learn that many modern procedures produce little or no discomfort.

Just as important, dentists are now much more aware of how their behavior and attitude shape the patient's experience. Many of today's dental education programs include coursework and lectures that address patient perceptions—the entire field fluorescent lights? Not in our practice. The light in our reception area and hallways is a calming dim yellow. While the professional staff requires bright wattage to do our jobs, the patient doesn't need that bright light, and so is given a pair of dark safety glasses as an option to cut back the glare. The glasses also create a sense of emotional safety and a symbolic barrier between the patient and the dental treatment.

We also take care to provide a calming aural environment. Put on your headphones and retreat into your own musical world, where Frank Sinatra is forever crooning those elegant standards, or Antonio Carlos Jobim is strumming out quiet chords from his bossa nova guitar. The only music you definitely won't hear in our office is the sound of me singing, and for that you can be grateful. Dr. Ted Goldstein, cofounder of a dental education program at Mt. Sinai Hospital in New York observes, "[Today] the dentist is trained to work slowly and to respect the patient's fear rather than deny it."

He couldn't be more right.

is changing to reflect these new sensitivities. Dentists realize that patients will take oral health more seriously if their anxiety levels are both acknowledged and addressed. As a result, dentists are taking steps to make the office experience as comfortable for the patient as possible. Massage therapy, hypnosis, biofeedback, and relaxation therapy are some of the measures being taken by dentists to help ease their patients. Today's dentists also recognize that one major cause of anxiety is lack of information, and are making a conscious effort to become better teachers when it comes to explaining care and treatment options.

If you haven't been to the dentist in a while, now is the time to begin anew. Schedule that long-overdue introductory appointment. Explain that you'd like to assess how comfortable you feel working with this practitioner. During this introductory visit, ask to see the dentist's equipment, and be sure the purpose of each unit is explained to you. Ask about the dentist's educational background including any special training.

No question is inappropriate. Mention your dental phobia and see how the dentist reacts. You might be surprised to find that he or she is used to dealing with this condition, and responds by providing information about treatment options. Your question should prompt a reply about methods the dentist uses to deal with patient fear of pain. If not, choose another dentist. (To learn more about finding the right dentist, see Chapter 2.)

If you feel comfortable with the practitioner, you might want to schedule a visit for a cleaning procedure before you leave the office. I recommend this because it's a tangible first step in overcoming the phobia that's undermined your oral health for years, and kept you from achieving the perfect smile.

THINGS TO REMEMBER

- Painful experiences in the dentist's chair during childhood can contribute to dental phobia later in life.

- There are different degrees of dental phobia. Most people are dental phobic to some degree.

- Fear of the dentist keeps many people from scheduling appointments on a regular basis. Oftentimes, their oral health deteriorates as a result.

- Dental phobia is often the product of selective memory. We forget the many dental sessions that passed without incident and remember only those visits when the drill really did hurt us.

- Only by acknowledging that you have dental phobia can you start to eliminate it.

- Many dentists these days are learning ways to combat patients' phobias, and there are a number who practice hypnosis, biofeedback, and other relaxation therapies.

Chapter 2

Choosing a Dentist

Making the Right Choice

Finding the dentist who is right for you is key to establishing and maintaining excellent oral health. It's a mistake to pick a practitioner out of the phone book or choose one solely on the basis of insurance coverage. The search for the right dentist might take some time and some effort. But the results—better health and progress toward the perfect smile—make it all worthwhile.

The best way to locate a good, reputable general dentist is by referral from a friend or family member. If you're seeking a specialist, try your family dentist for the best referral.

But what if you don't have a regular dentist? Perhaps you've relocated recently to a new neighborhood, your prior practitioner has retired, or like many Americans, you've simply put off going to the dentist for so long that you realize you don't actually have a dentist.

Of course, it's entirely possible that you don't fall into any of these categories. It's conceivable that you have a skilled dentist committed to his or her patients and that you are delighted with the quality of care he or she provides. Of course, in that case, I don't recommend that you blithely switch practitioners simply for the sake of change.

Whether or not you're satisfied with your current dentist, reading this chapter should raise some interesting questions for you to consider. You may realize that your current dentist is in fact the best choice for you. Conversely, you might decide it's time to do some research and find the dentist who's best equipped to help you with your present needs.

It's important to mention that individual preferences play a large part in what is, in the end, a very personal choice. The dentist who has treated your neighbor for twenty years and "walks on water" as far as your neighbor is concerned might be entirely wrong for you. It isn't necessarily a question of competence, but one of style, interpersonal dynamics, and suitability for particular health needs. Nevertheless, asking your neighbor for a referral is an ideal place to start your search. After all, a fine dentist will generate great word of mouth.

You might also ask for referrals from others who have steered you right in the past. Consider consulting coworkers, cousins, your pastor, your gym workout buddy, your fellow fire department volunteers—anyone whose judgment you trust and who lives or works within a reasonable distance of the dentist's office.

Finally, surfing the Web will introduce you to a myriad of dental sites and directories (see *Resources*). These sites offer information on various dental procedures as well as lists of local dentists. Remember to examine specific qualifications like special experience and teaching appointments—and don't forget to consider how convenient the dentist's location is to your home or work. When you ask for a referral, ask some or all of the following questions.

- How long have you been treated by Dr. _____?
- How did you learn about Dr. _____?
- Is insurance coverage your main consideration?
- How helpful are the hygienist and other office personnel?
- Why did you change from your previous dentist?
- How long does it take to get an appointment with Dr. _____?
- What is Dr. _____'s best quality as a dentist?
- What, if anything, about Dr. _____'s practice annoys you?

These questions all call for subjective answers, and that's the point. Your neighbor's criteria might be—and probably are—different from yours. For example, insurance coverage may factor heavily in some people's decisions, whereas others might have particular health requirements or scheduling needs to consider. Speak with people you trust and you'll quickly see just how subjective the entire process truly is.

You might also develop your own list of questions before beginning your search. They should clearly reflect your particular needs, circumstances, preferences, health history, treatment aversions, and so on. It is okay to be subjective—It's your health, and your money. You're entitled to be as particular as you please. To determine your preferences as a patient, you might consider which of the following issues are important to you. (Not all will be, of course.)

Practitioner style. Do you prefer a dentist who is friendly and extremely solicitous, asking about your comfort at every step, or do you prefer a brisk practitioner who proceeds on the assumption that if you're uncomfortable you'll express that?

Appointment availability. Are you restricted to certain days of the week or certain times of the day when scheduling appointments? Can the dentist accommodate your schedule?

Office location. Is the practitioner's office conveniently located near where you live or work, or will you have to go out of your way to get there?

Appointment reliability. Some dentists adhere to schedules more than others. Some even schedule several patients for the same time slot. Can you afford to wait half an hour, or would that be a problem for you?

Expertise. If you have particular procedures in mind, such as cosmetic dentistry or implant tooth replacement, does the practitioner have adequate experience in that specialty? How many years has he or she been treating patients with this specialized care?

Financial considerations. Money is the first thing that many patients—and practitioners—want to discuss.

Insurance plan coverage. You should have no difficulty learning from the dentist's office staff whether or not they accept your insurance plan. Keep in mind, however, that many plans provide only partial coverage for many procedures, and may limit the frequency of procedures that are covered in full. For instance, your plan might pay for two cleanings a year but your dentist may recommend three.

It isn't enough to learn only whether your plan covers a particular practitioner. You will also need to ask whether the office requires full payment up front or accepts a co-payment—usually in the $10 to $25 range—and handles its own reimbursement. (If it doesn't, you are expected to pay the full amount, then file paperwork yourself to receive reimbursement.)

Keep in mind that insurance coverage fluctuates enormously. Insurance companies frequently change their policies in connection with reimbursement rates, co-payment amounts, scheduling, and the like. Practitioners also feel little obligation to remain "loyal" to plans that themselves have no loyalty. It isn't unusual for a dentist to start out working with numerous insurers and then, years later, begin weeding out the more difficult payers, or simply dropping coverage altogether. For this reason, searching for a dentist based primarily on insurance coverage is not recommended.

You should also ask about alternative payment methods. Many dentists still follow the traditional policy of requiring payment in full at the end of each visit. In fact, many dentists today are choosing to switch from insurance-based practices to a fee-for-service system to regain control over treatment processes and patient care.

More and more dentists offer flexible payment policies, even for more complicated procedures. Ask whether the office can work out a monthly payment schedule rather than up-front payment. Some offices accept credit cards, too. Your dentist should not make you feel in any way embarrassed for asking questions about the fee structure or payment policies. When recommending any treatment plan your dentist should be willing to specify fee structure and schedules (and be willing to put it in writing.)

Warrantees. Few dentists guarantee their work for a specified time period, so a practitioner who offers an approximate time period, and refuses to put the guarantee in writing, is not necessarily inferior. However, a dentist who does stand behind his work is undoubtedly confident of its lasting quality. That certainly is a good sign, though the patient should also understand that much dental work is time-limited. Your dentist should alert you to the life span of the treatment rendered and what he or she recommends if the work needs to be redone at some later date, as it often does.

Lastly, consider **comparison shopping.** We live in a free market, which means dentists—like lawyers, electricians and house painters—can charge what the market will bear. As a result, fees vary considerably. The dentist who charges the highest fees is not necessarily the best dentist, nor is the one who charges the lowest fees the worst. *Consumer Research* magazine surveyed 439 dentists in the Washington, D.C., area in the mid-1990s and found that fees for procedures such as single root canal and crown varied by as much as $520. The study also found there was no correlation between the dentist's fee and patient satisfaction with the quality of care.

Non-Fee Criteria

Office cleanliness. This is nonnegotiable. Waiting and treatment rooms, as well as the patient's bathroom, should be immaculate. A dentist who doesn't insist on spotless surroundings in the patient areas is likely to care little about the cleanliness of what you can't see.

Equipment sterilization. All equipment and instruments used in patient care should be sterilized in accordance with professional guidelines outlined by the Occupational Safety & Health Administration (OSHA) after each use to avoid transfer of diseases between patients. Every dentist should have—and use—an autoclave, chemical vapor, or dry heat oven. Don't be afraid to ask about sterilization techniques at your dentist's office.

Personal Anti-Contagion Precautions. Beginning in the 1980s, the threat of AIDS transmission motivated most dentists and hygienists to wear rubber gloves, mouth masks, and eye goggles when treating patients. Government requirements have since made such precautions nearly universal, and have eliminated the

Finding Hidden Cavities with Technology

Dental technology has come a long way since the old days when the dentist would probe around your mouth with a mirror looking for cavities. These days, your dentist can locate hidden decay before it destroys the tooth structure from the inside out. The tool she uses is called a DIAGNOdent. It's a small laser instrument that scans the teeth with harmless, painless laser light and detects cavities too small to see with the naked eye. That allows your dentist to spot and repair small cavities before they grow to big ones.

risk of dental contagion from blood-borne diseases like AIDS or hepatitis. You should absolutely avoid using a practitioner who does not strictly adhere to these precautions.

Group or solo practice. It is tempting to conclude that a dentist who belongs to a group practice draws from a wide array of resources, casually consults colleagues on knotty issues, and utilizes the availability of partners who can fill in during an emergency. While logical, that conclusion can be erroneous. Most patients say the care received from a dentist practicing in a group differs little if at all from a dentist practicing solo.

Credentials. Every dentist must be licensed by the state to practice, and must complete approximately 25 hours of continuing education every 2 years for license renewal. (The number of hours varies by state.) Unfortunately, the license does not

Understanding Dental Specialties

Here's a breakdown of the leading dental specialties.

- **Endodontist:** Handles difficult root canal treatment.
- **Oral surgeon:** Removes impacted teeth, performs various jaw surgeries, and surgically places dental implants.
- **Orthodontist:** Straightens multiple teeth, utilizing braces or other devices.
- **Periodontist:** Treats advanced gum and periodontal disease, gum surgery, and the surgical placement of dental implants.
- **Prosthodontist:** Provides the restoration, beautification, and/or replacement of teeth.

guarantee quality of care and should not be interpreted as such. Nor does the license imply that the dentist has been subjected to peer review.

Up-to-date equipment. There are dentists who have not updated their equipment in more than a decade. Equipment developed in recent years has greatly enhanced the profession, and brought great benefits to many patients. Your dentist should not have obsolete equipment. Consider asking your doctor: What's the newest equipment in your office, and how can it help me?

Communication style. Does your dentist provide you with an emergency phone number (and if you call, do you get a response?) Does your dentist give out his e-mail address?

Celebrity status. This criterion wouldn't have been mentioned a few years ago, but we live in an era of celebrity adulation. There are now celebrity lawyers, celebrity doctors, even, celebrity dentists. I would not advise choosing a dentist because you saw his or her face in the newspapers or on television. This could be as a result of a good publicist or a personal connection with the reporter. On the other hand, if you do see your dentist on TV, definitely mention it the next time you sit down in his or her chair. Dentists have egos too.

Specialization. Most (but not all) dentists who decide to specialize seek additional professional education and board certification in their specialties. They usually list their certifications and affiliations on their business cards or office informational material.

Evaluating Quality of Care

You could say that choosing a dentist is a little like getting married; you never really know what you're in for until after the wedding. You can interview a dentist and ask all the right questions, and not really be sure if the match will work until after you've sat in the chair. If you're not happy with a specific aspect of your provider's care, you should speak up, and explain what you would like done differently.

Here are some questions to ask yourself when evaluating your present practitioner and the quality of his or her work.

- Does Dr. _____ ask about oral health problems? Your dentist should ask questions about your oral health, specifically about procedures performed in past visits and whether the treatment successfully ended the symptoms. He or she should also follow up on problems mentioned in previous visits. Your dentist should maintain charts tracking your treatment history and refer to them while you're in the chair.

- Does Dr. _____ or an assistant discuss routine dental hygiene? Most people have flawed brushing and flossing techniques. Studies have shown a reduction in the incidence of periodontal disease and the rate of tooth decay in patients of dentists who offer periodic brushing and flossing demonstrations, and correct patients after observing their brushing techniques.

- Does Dr. _____'s office staff provide professional service? Are they helpful? Most importantly, are they able to schedule appointments when you need them?

- Did Dr. _____ take a thorough history at the initial exam? Did he or she ask about allergies or reactions to certain drugs that might be used in treatment, and about current medication use? Did he or she ask to see copies of recent x-rays, or recommend taking a full set of x-rays if no recent images were available?

- Does Dr. _____ offer digitized radiographs (x-rays)?

- Did Dr. ___ provide you with a lead apron if x-rays were taken?

- Did Dr. _____ probe your gums, specifically the pockets between teeth and gums?

- Did Dr. _____ check your mouth for the warning signs of oral cancer?

- Did Dr. _____ explain the procedures, or did he or she presume you understood them and approved? If you objected to a procedure, or asked that it be postponed, did the doctor suggest alternative treatments, or probe your resistance?

- Did Dr. _____ offer you informational material when recommending a procedure, and if so was the material written or communicated in plain English? Was he or she available to discuss the information in the brochures or video?

- Did Dr. _____ tailor the treatment to you and your particular requirements? Your health needs and lifestyle should determine the treatment schedule and procedures. A good dentist does not apply one-size-fits-all policies, but rather suggests that certain patients come in more often for cleanings, if for example, a predilection for gum disease is noted.

- Perhaps most importantly, did Dr. _____ provide treatment that produced the desired results? Were you able to close your mouth properly after your visit? Keep in mind that treatment might not cure or eliminate all the problems involved. In such cases, treatment options should be discussed. You might want to prompt your dentist for a referral to a specialist.

- Did Dr. _____ cause you repeated discomfort during treatment? With all the new anesthetics and technology available today, consistent discomfort during treatment could be a warning sign. If your visits seem unusually painful or cumbersome, consider changing dentists.

Dentists are hardworking and dedicated health professionals. If you're unhappy with your present practitioner, follow your instinct and find a different dentist. But before making the switch, try to convey your feelings about the quality of care to your doctor. Dentists aren't mind readers and do a better job when patients communicate honestly. If you're dissatisfied, let your dentist know, and explain why. And if you're pleased, make sure to thank your practitioner.

THINGS TO REMEMBER

- A good way to find a reputable general dentist is by referral from a friend or family member. But keep in mind that a dentist who's right for a coworker or friend may not necessarily be right for you.

- If you're looking for a specialist, consult your family dentist for a referral.

- Some important factors to consider when choosing a dentist include the practitioner's style and expertise, the availability of appointments that suit your schedule, the location of the office, and financial matters such as fees and insurance coverage.

- Important features to pay attention to include the dentist's credentials, care in sterilizing equipment, personal anti-contagion precautions, communication style, specialization, and the overall cleanliness of the office.

- You should feel free to comparison shop for a dentist who will provide you with quality care at appropriate fees.

- Communicate with your dentist. If something dissatisfies you, let your dentist know—dentists aren't mind readers!

Cosmetic Options

The State of the Art

The term cosmetic dentistry is misleading. The word *cosmetic* implies a superficial, temporary change—like applying makeup. But cosmetic dentistry is neither superficial nor short-term, and includes a combination of dental treatments that change the way you look and feel.

On the other hand, the term does convey some important realities. The dictionary defines cosmetic primarily as something "used to beautify," and secondarily as "tending to improve facial or physical attractiveness." Cosmetic dentistry whitens what time has yellowed, eliminates gaps where small spaces once prevailed, and smoothes what has become chipped and uneven. Although not a fountain of youth, an investment in cosmetic dentistry can have a tremendous effect on your appearance, and consequently, on how others respond to you.

People sometimes imply that cosmetic dentistry is a frivolous indulgence in vanity. But it's undeniable that we're often initially judged on the basis of appearance, and that a large part of our appearance is our smile. First impressions matter—and often have lasting effects.

Most successful people value basic grooming and good hygiene. Each morning, and perhaps again in the evening, they wash their face, comb their hair, shave or apply makeup, and check the mirror. To go out without having completed this series of routine tasks is to risk social embarrassment. We've all seen people who look like they've just gotten out of bed—their hair a rat's nest of tangled locks, shirts flapping, dots of shaving cream behind their ear. We wonder: "Doesn't this poor soul own a mirror?"

Although other people's shortcomings seem glaringly obvious, it's human nature to overlook our own deficiencies, and presume others are equally forgiving. Just this once, take a closer look at what others see when you smile at them in greeting. You've washed up, you smell great, you've brushed your hair, clipped or painted your fingernails, and smoothed your jacket. You feel pretty good about yourself. You're ready to take on the world, and the world doesn't stand a chance. You gaze at the mirror and say: Everything is fantastic.

But is it?

Let's take a close, candid, and unflinching look at the face you're preparing to show the world. Stand in front of the mirror, look at your mouth, and smile. Now, lean forward a bit, draw back your gums, and grin. Look carefully in the mirror. After grinding several tons of food during your lifetime, the surfaces of your teeth have become uneven, and some may be chipped. You've also consumed a river of beverages over the years—coffee, wine, tea, and cola have stained your teeth yellow, brown, and black. Are you a smoker, or even a former smoker? Then it's likely all those cigarettes, cigars, or pipes have left behind yellow-brown nicotine residue. All those times you failed to brush your gums have left them a little puffy and loose around the teeth. Your teeth have shifted slightly over the years and now jut out in jagged discolored protrusions.

The truth is, after a few decades our mouths start to show the effects of all that wear and tear. Our smile does not look very appealing. We smile less often, showing fewer teeth and even less self-confidence.

Our attitude of dental self-delusion stands in marked contrast to how many of us deal with other physical shortcomings. We go to the gym and work out to keep our abs looking good, diet to lessen that potbelly, and get fitted for contact lenses to do away with the heavy glasses. We shop for Rogaine in hopes of getting back our full head of hair. What about our teeth? Aside from twice-a-year cleanings, many choose to simply tolerate the awful shape of their mouths.

In the past, this fatalistic attitude towards dental health might have been understandable. Our parents' generation had few alternatives. Unless you were a Hollywood star or some other high net worth individual whose livelihood depended on scheduled flashing of those pearly whites, you tolerated the deplorable condition of your teeth and gums. Except for the very wealthy, dental treatment was limited to repairing the damage done by decay.

Today it's a different story. Cosmetic dentistry is no longer the expensive, time-consuming and burdensome process of yesteryear. Consequently, millions of people have made the decision to upgrade their smiles.

Cosmetic dentistry is one of the fastest growing areas of the field. In a recent survey, the American Academy of Cosmetic Dentistry found that the number of people who underwent tooth whitening or bleaching procedures more than tripled in the second half of the 1990s. The popularity of other forms of cosmetic dentistry has also skyrocketed, with the decrease in cost and discomfort levels, and the increase in public acceptance.

In the rest of this chapter, we'll survey the major options available to those who have decided to invest in beautifying their smiles.

Filling Options

Until fairly recently in the history of tooth repair, fillings were available in two varieties: gold alloy or silver amalgam. Each of these compounds has a proven record of success and durability, and both are still widely used today. However, newer materials that closely resemble natural tooth color have become available in recent years; you might consider one of them if you have concerns about your smile and appearance.

As with other dental treatments, the decision about what to fill your cavities with is best made in consultation with your dentist, and should take into account your individual situation—the size and location of the cavity, your medical history, cosmetic concerns, degree of insurance coverage.

Ceramic materials. Ceramic materials are an important option to consider. They're appropriate for filling cavities, repairing chipped teeth, and covering discolored tooth enamel. Ceramic restorations are highly resistant to wear, but require at least two visits to the dentist, and usually cost more than other types of restorations. All-porcelain restorations have particular appeal for many because their color and translucency closely mimic natural tooth enamel, but they have a tendency to fracture under tension. For this reason, many opt for combined porcelain and metal restorations,

The Truth About Amalgam Fillings

Silver-colored fillings, known as dental amalgam, have been the subject of much debate recently. It is true that amalgam contains mercury, but when it is mixed with metals such as silver, copper, and tin, it forms a stable alloy that dentists have used for years to successfully treat dental disease in millions of people.

In the same way that sodium and chlorine (both hazardous in their pure state) combine to form ordinary table salt, the mercury in dental amalgam combines with other metals to form a stable dental filling. Amalgam, like all other dental filling materials currently in use, is safe and effective. In fact, the Food and Drug Administration (FDA), Centers for Disease Control and Prevention (CDCP), U.S. Public Health Service (USPHS), National Institutes of Health (NIH) and the World Health Organization (WHO), have extensively evaluated amalgam time and time again and declared it safe and effective.

which are very durable and strong.

Tooth-colored fillings or bonding. Tooth-colored fillings (also known as bonding) are made from a resin called composite, used to fill in small cavities or chips. Bonding eliminates the metallic look that characterizes the mouths of many baby boomers, who grew up in a time when cavities were frequent occurrences. Until well into the 1990s, most fillings were made of a composite medium with a mercury base. People who feel self-

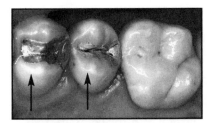

Two gold alloy fillings

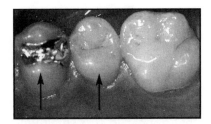

One gold alloy and one
tooth-colored filling

conscious about all that silver in their smile are now opting to replace those fillings with resin, when the cavities are small enough to make this permissible. Resin can become discolored over time, but the initial cost is usually cheaper than a porcelain restoration.

Of the two methods for applying resin composite fillings, the direct method is fastest. Your dentist removes the decay from your tooth and applies the resin in one session. In the case of the indirect method, your dentist makes an impression of your tooth and sends it to a lab that fabricates a restoration; the restoration is then bonded or cemented in place. These laboratory heat-processed restorations tend to last longer than the direct in-office white fillings, but are considerably more expensive.

Recontouring Your Smile

Gingivectomy. Recontouring is one of the most important developments of cosmetic dentistry. Very often cosmetic recontouring involves a gingivectomy, or "gum lift," in which the dentist removes the patient's excess gum tissue. The procedure usually takes not more than half an hour per tooth.

Have you noticed that when some people smile they seem to reveal too much gum, or their teeth appear to be uneven in length? This condition can be hereditary. Other times it is the result of gradual softening of the gums with age—especially after years of failing to brush the gums vigorously (this applies to the teeth as well.)

A gingivectomy is the dental equivalent of liposuction, producing major aesthetic benefits quickly. Your smile will be softer and less gummy—more of your teeth will be visible. Teeth that appeared too small will look larger and more attractive.

Tooth reshaping. Another kind of recontouring is tooth reshaping. This involves scraping off a wafer-thin slice of enamel from your tooth to remove uneven or chipped edges

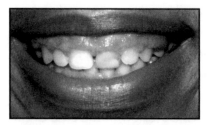 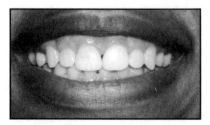

Before gingivectomy and laminates   **After** gingivectomy and laminates

or other imperfections. This process can shorten teeth that seem too long and round teeth that have become pointed. Since enamel has no nerve connections, you will feel no pain as your dentist sculpts a more attractive smile.

Laminates. We call this "veneering" the perfect smile. Individuals who feel their teeth are misshapen, discolored, chipped, or somehow unattractive are delighted with this affordable solution to oral disfigurement.

Here's how it works: After minimal tooth preparation involving the removal of enamel, the dentist takes an impression of the front of the tooth and creates a very thin porcelain veneer, which is then glued in place. This is essentially half a crown, covering only the front surface and edge of the tooth, protecting it and improving its appearance. This is often the best solution when a full crown is not needed.

The process usually takes two to three visits. Your dentist sends the impression to a dental laboratory that fabricates the laminate. You can expect your porcelain veneer to last 10 to 15 years, depending on your home care, regular hygiene visits to your dentist, and the relative gentleness with which you treat the veneer.

Your tooth might feel a little different for a week or two, and then you'll grow accustomed to your new "pearly whites."

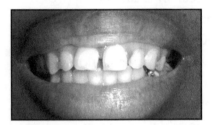 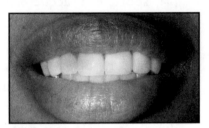

Before laminates   **After** laminates

The satisfaction rate is high; most patients who receive porcelain veneers are delighted with their new appearance. Next to tooth whitening, porcelain veneers or laminates are the most frequently requested cosmetic treatment in the United States.

Tooth Whitening

Yellow teeth are particularly noticeable and stigmatizing, especially when you otherwise appear youthful and healthy. Overcoming this very visible sign of aging has been the work of dentists for many generations. Tooth whitening (or bleaching) is the least invasive—and least expensive—way to brighten your teeth. Understandably, tooth whitening has become the most common medical or dental cosmetic procedure in the United States today.

Fast Facts About Porcelain Veneers

Results: Can fix one imperfect tooth or give you an entirely new smile.

Upkeep: Avoid prescription-grade fluoride, which can stain, and stop the fingernail biting, which can chip or crack the porcelain. If you tend to grind your teeth or play sports like racquetball, soccer, or basketball, a professional mouth guard is recommended.

Cost: From $1,200 to $2,000 per tooth, depending on the difficulty of your case as well as the education and experience of the dentist and ceramist.

Advantages: Long-lasting results; noninvasive procedure; virtually instant gratification. No long-term orthodontics required.

Disadvantages: Won't last forever; potential for initial sensitivity. As you age, non-treated teeth will yellow naturally and may have to be bleached to match. Not reversible; not permanent.

Endurance: Can last 8 to 12 years.

There are two ways to have your teeth whitened: Do it yourself at home or have the procedure performed by your dentist.

At-home whitening. There are several types of products available for use at home—some are dispensed by your dentist, while others can be purchased over-the-counter.

Bleaching solutions contain peroxide, which actually bleaches tooth enamel. The bleaching agent in these products is usually

Talk to Your Dentist About Tooth Whitening

If you're considering tooth whitening you may want to start by speaking with your dentist. He or she can tell you whether such procedures would be effective for you. Whiteners may not correct all types of discoloration. For example, yellow-ish hued teeth will probably bleach well, brownish-colored teeth may bleach less well, and grayish-hued teeth may not bleach at all. Likewise, bleaching may not enhance your smile if you have had bonding or tooth-colored fillings placed in your front teeth. The whitener will not affect the color of these materials, and they will stand out in your newly whitened smile. In these cases, you may want to investigate alternatives like porcelain veneers or dental bonding.

carbamide peroxide, which is available in 10, 16, and 22 percent concentrations.

Whiteners that contain peroxide typically come in gel form and are placed in a mouthguard. Some products are used twice a day for 2 weeks, and others are intended for overnight use for a 1- to 2-week period. If you obtain the bleaching solution from your dentist, he or she can construct a custom mouth guard to fit your teeth precisely. Currently, only dentist-dispensed home-use 10 percent carbamide peroxide tray-applied gels carry the American Dental Association (ADA) seal.

Speak with your dentist if any side effects become bothersome. For example, teeth can become sensitive during the

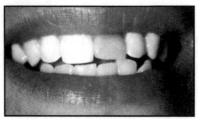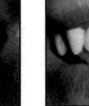

Before laminates and tooth reshaping   **After** laminates and tooth reshaping

period when you are using the bleaching solution. In many cases, this sensitivity is temporary and should lessen once the treatment is finished. Some people also experience soft tissue irritation—either from a tray that doesn't fit properly or from solution that may come in contact with soft tissue. If you have concerns about such side effects, you should discuss them with your dentist.

Toothpastes help remove surface stain through the action of mild abrasives. "Whitening" toothpastes in the ADA Seal of Acceptance program have special chemical or polishing agents that provide additional stain removal effectiveness. Unlike bleaches, these ADA accepted products do not alter the intrinsic color of teeth.

When selecting a whitener or any dental product, be sure to look for the ADA Seal of Acceptance. This seal is your assurance that the product has met ADA standards of safety and effectiveness.

In-Office Whitening. Although tooth whitening is easy to do at home, results may not be evident for up to six weeks, provided the teeth are treated daily. For this reason, some patients choose to speed up the process by having the procedure done by their dentist.

For more than a century, dentists have used hydrogen peroxide to whiten stained teeth. With the advent of potent agents like carbamide peroxide in recent years, the efficacy of in-office whitenings has increased dramatically. The peroxide gel is placed into a custom-fitted tray in your mouth, and works by releasing free radicals that attack years of stains and discoloration on your teeth.

The results of this process are often extraordinary, so much so that previous restorations in your mouth will appear discolored. To avoid such an occurrence, select tooth-colored restorations that match your newly-whitened teeth to replace earlier work. This way, your new smile will look uniform.

Power bleaching is now rapidly becoming the tooth whitening treatment of choice. Some individuals with severe discoloration, or those who want to see quick results, are candidates for this approach, which uses the highest concentrated form of hydrogen peroxide to produce the most profound whitening. In this procedure, the dentist applies a high intensity light to trigger the reaction of hydrogen peroxide on your teeth. Special methods are used to isolate the teeth being bleached and protect the gum tissue and cheeks from the powerful bleaching agents used. Results are noticeable before you leave the office.

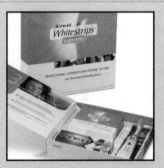

Photo © Crest

Whitening strips are among the newest at-home tooth-whitening products. Crest Whitestrips Supreme (shown at left) are one such product sold in retail stores. The flexible, invisible strips are coated with an enamel-safe tooth bleaching gel. You place the strips on your teeth and wear them for a specified number of minutes. After 21 days, your teeth will be whiter and brighter.

Several visits are generally required, depending on the severity of the discoloration and the degree of whiteness desired. Also note that the treatment does not produce permanent results. If you maintain exemplary oral hygiene habits—refrain from cigarettes, coffee, tea, cola, and red wine—your newly-bleached teeth should stay white longer. Otherwise, you may decide to repeat the procedure at a later date.

Straightening Your Teeth

Malocclusions, or "bad bites," are very common, and fortunately quite easy to fix. Frequently the product of tooth crowding, malocclusions affect your smile and appearance, and may interfere with your ability to floss. Oftentimes, braces are a simple and very effective way to move your teeth into their appropriate positions and fix the overall shape of your bite. Braces are not just for kids anymore; in fact, they're now an appealing solution for people of all ages. It is never too late to improve your smile.

The first step toward correcting a malocclusion is to ask your dentist for a reference to an orthodontist. Orthodontists are specialists trained to deal with irregularities of the teeth. To obtain an accurate diagnosis and decide

David M. Momtaheni, D.M.D, President of the American Society for Lasers in Medicine and Advanced Technology for Dentistry states that the FDA has recently approved some lasers for hard tissue use, meaning for removal of minimal to moderate dental decay. Also, two types of dental lasers—the argon and the CO_2—have been approved for use in teeth bleaching. The latter was designed specifically for whitening deeper tooth stains.

on the plan of treatment that is best for you, the orthodontist may take x-rays of your mouth or a plaster cast of your teeth and gums. He or she will then construct a custom-fitted appliance that will correct the specific problems in your bite. Brackets are then bonded to your teeth with a wire running between them. Throughout the course of your treatment, your braces are adjusted periodically so that your teeth move gradually into place.

The exact time required for braces to correct tooth alignment varies from person to person, but it is usually around 2 years. Adults may take a little longer to treat, but many feel the results are worth it. If you've been thinking about correcting your bite, but have concerns about your appearance during treatment, several less noticeable options are now available. The brackets that hold the wires in place can be translucent or tooth colored. Some people even opt for braces in the back of their teeth, depending on the kind of correction required.

While there is no question that braces are expensive, millions of children and adults continue to opt for appliances that will fix their bites. Many feel that the cost and slight inconvenience more than justify the end results—a beautiful smile to be proud of.

The popular procedures we've just discussed are only some of the ways in which dentistry is helping people obtain the perfect smile. Dentistry continues to evolve, and progress is made everyday on this front. By the time you finish reading this book, new procedures might well have become mainstream practice!

THINGS TO REMEMBER

• Cosmetic dentistry is no longer the time-consuming and expensive process it once was. Many people have made the decision to improve their smiles in recent years. It's one of the fastest growing areas in the field.

• A procedure called a gingivectomy, or "gum lift," will soften your smile by removing excess gum tissue. Other options are available to reshape teeth and smooth away chipped edges and imperfections.

• Many people these days have bonding applied to their teeth and opt for tooth colored filings to replace the silver in their smiles.

• "Veneering" is an affordable solution for many types of tooth disfigurement and discoloration.

• Tooth whitening has become the most popular medical procedure in the United States. At-home options are available as are in-office treatments.

• Braces aren't just for kids anymore. People of all ages are discovering how braces can help them achieve the perfect smile.

Chapter 4

Tooth Replacement

A Second Chance

Losing a tooth isn't an uncommon experience. The Centers for Disease Control and Prevention report that seven out of 10 adults between ages 35 and 44 have lost at least one permanent tooth. By age 50, the average American has lost 12 teeth. More than one-quarter of those ages 65 to 74 have lost all their teeth.

Whether caused by tooth decay, periodontal disease, or physical trauma, losing teeth has both physiological and emotional consequences. From the physiological perspective, chewing becomes difficult. The individual begins to avoid certain foods. This (usually unplanned) dietary change results in a compromised health regimen.

The most significant damage, however, is often to self-esteem. When we cannot smile proudly we tend to retreat into ourselves—avoiding interaction, going out less often, and meeting fewer people.

There are a number of traditional solutions to the problem of missing teeth. Dental rehabilitation, or restorative dentistry, is one of the fastest-growing specialties in dentistry today. Techniques and prostheses have both improved, and more dentists are aware of the great impact implants have on people's lives. If you have lost one or more teeth, there are a number of options available to you.

One of the options is bridgework. There are in fact two types of bridgework: removable and fixed.

Test Tube Teeth?

Did you know that by age 50 most Americans have lost an average of 12 teeth? Poor dental hygiene and periodontal disease claim billions of teeth each year, keeping scientists busy looking for new ways to replace them. In September 2002, a research team led by Pamela C. Yelick, PhD at the Forsyth Dental Institute in Boston announced they were able to isolate tooth cells from young pigs and grow them into fully formed teeth. Though the research is still in its early stages, it seems to suggest the existence of dental stem cells, which have enormous potential in many areas of tooth repair, experts say. Maybe someday when our pearly whites go, we'll simply be able to grow a new set in a test tube.

Removable Dentures

The removable or partial denture is a set of artificial teeth that must come out at bedtime. Generally made of plastic or cast metal, dentures are custom-fitted to match and adhere to the upper or lower jaw or to clamp onto remaining original teeth through metal supports known as clasps.

While many learn to live with dentures, the solution is imperfect at best . The lower jaw, called the mandible, is particularly difficult to fit. It is important to note that even if the dentures are well fitted, not everyone adjusts well to them. People often complain that wearing dentures, especially at the beginning, makes them feel like gagging. Additionally, a process known as residual ridge resorption causes jawbone shrinkage, so denture fit tends to loosen over time. This requires the wearer to schedule follow-up visits so the dentist can do a refitting, known as a reline.

Another problem is that the pressure exerted by dentures on the gums, or flange, can cause sores. People often complain that dentures are uncomfortable, and liken the feeling to pancakes getting stuck to the roof of the mouth or around the tongue. This problem is compounded by the fact that many people put off scheduling the necessary follow-up visits. Consequently, it's not surprising that denture wearing seems to be one of life's more uncomfortable accommodations.

Permanent Teeth

When dentures (aka bridges) are made permanent they are called fixed bridges. One of the advantages of having a fixed bridge installed is that it remains stationary. You can hold a conversation or eat a meal without worrying that your teeth will move.

Irwin Smigel, President Emeritus of the American Society for Dental Aesthetics, told the *Ladies Home Journal* recently, "A fixed bridge is less likely than a removable one to irritate the gums and trap plaque. It's also more comfortable, easier to chew with and, psychologically, far more satisfying."[1]

Artificial Teeth

For a more permanent solution many people choose to have artificial teeth (usually porcelain) affixed to their adjacent teeth. To make the artificial tooth, the dentist files down the neighboring teeth, takes a mold, and sends it to a dental laboratory, where the replacement teeth (including the two adjacent teeth) are fabricated. The artificial teeth are then cemented in place by the dentist.

Because bridges tend to damage the surrounding teeth, in recent years tooth replacements have been fabricated using resin or metal "wings" to minimize impact on adjacent teeth.

Because this process requires neighboring teeth to be healthy, it's not ideal for every patient. In addition, some dentists discourage bridgework because it adds stress to adjacent teeth and may cause them to become unstable. Over years of use, the stress can result in the bridge bond loosening. Bridgework therefore is not truly a permanent solution.

The Dental Implant

Advances in dental implants offer enormous hope for people who have lost teeth. In fact, the number of such procedures tripled during the 1990s, according to the American Dental Association. The procedure is technically known as an endosseous implant. The implant behaves like an artificial root on top of which a new artificial porcelain tooth can later be screwed in or cemented. The implant is inserted surgically in the existing jawbone and can remain in place for years. The procedure to place the implant is a minor, two-step surgical process. While some people express concern at undergoing minor surgery, the procedure is actually less invasive than having a tooth removed. There is another significant, therapeutic benefit to implants: They prevent further bone loss and help maintain ridge form.

A brief history. About 50 years ago, dentists began using an implant that required the insertion of a blade-like device into the bone of the jaw. However, the blade did not fuse to the bone, and required tissue to grow around it.

In the mid-1960s, in Sweden, a pioneering orthopedic surgeon, Per-Ingvar Branemark, experimented and made a major discovery. He dramatically improved the success rate of implants by milling the root-shaped implant from titanium, which the body accepts as a natural substance. The bone grows right up to the implant and bonds with it, forming an osseointegrated biological seal. It was Branemark who coined the term osseointegration.

Recent developments. In recent years the development of new techniques and the introduction of new materials have made implants state-of-the-art for tooth replacement. There have been major advances in the form of the materials that coat the screw, the design or surface topography of the screw, and in engineering the interface between screw and artificial tooth.

"Implants are much better designed than they used to be," Dr. Martha Somerman, president of the American Association for Dental Research, told The New York Times. "Individual implants today are quite successful. However, the success depends on the integrity of the patients' own bone, and the ability to build new bone if needed."[2]

Further experiments determined that certain titanium alloys are also accepted by the body, and today, pure titanium is gener-

Overdenture Prosthesis

ally used. It is light and noncorrosive and seems to be the most predictable material for implant construction. Titanium alloys, though, are not uncommon.

Implants are also used to anchor dentures. Small titanium buttons are placed in incisions in the roof of the mouth and connected to the gum side of the denture. As a result, dentures fit better, are less likely to shift in the mouth, and remain in place over longer periods.

What is the Implant Treatment Process Like?

The first step in receiving implants is an oral examination, which often includes dental x-rays or CT scans, to determine the quality and quantity of the bone in the areas that will support the implants. In some cases, after examining the potential implant sites, the practitioner recommends minor surgical procedures to expand bone mass or bone grafting to accommodate the implants, if warranted.

One such procedure is *sinus augmentation,* or sinus "lift." In this procedure, the sinus floor of the upper back jaw is raised to add volume and height.

Another procedure is *ridge modification.* Here the surgeon grafts bone or bone substitute onto the jaw. (This has the fortunate side effect of correcting any facial deformity.)

Most dental implants are one- or two-stage cylindrical implants, and can be done at a hospital or dentist's office using local anesthesia.

The first stage of the most common implant treatment

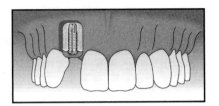

Osseointegrated anchor

involves surgically drilling screws into the jawbone to anchor the artificial tooth or teeth. In two-stage implants, a cylinder is inserted into the bone of the jaw. After allowing the gum to heal for seven to 10 days, the patient can resume his or her usual diet. The *osseointegration,* bonding between the implant and the jawbone, takes place over the next three to six months. Four to six months later, the site is reopened and the dentist screws in a small metal cap or abutment that connects the prosthetic tooth to the anchor.

In either case, two to four weeks later, after the gums have healed, the restorative dentist applies porcelain crowns or a fixed bridge to each extension. This part of the process usually requires several appointments over a period of one to two months, though some cases can take longer.

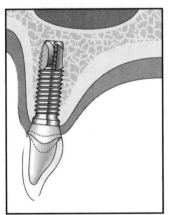

Osseointegraed anchor with artificial tooth

Hans-Peter Weber, writing in the *Harvard Health Letter,* said the process works very well, most of the time. "If patients are properly selected and evaluated, complications such as nerve damage, bone loss or fracture, or injury to healthy teeth are rare. The chance that an implanted fixture will crack or break off is less than one in a thousand. As with any surgical procedure, of course, infections and other healing problems may occur."[3]

He added this caveat: "Although reliable statistics are not available, aesthetic complications are probably more common. Patients may not like the looks of their new teeth because, for example, a bit of hardware is visible when they smile broadly. And sometimes people's speech changes, particularly when they begin wearing the prosthesis and when the upper jaw is involved. It is very important to discuss these issues with the dentist before starting treatment."[4]

Are implants right for you? Not everyone is a candidate for implants. Conditions that can rule out dental implants include alcohol, drug, or tobacco abuse, diabetes, bone deterioration, and bruxism (habitual tooth grinding). The procedure is advised with caution for individuals who have had joint replacement, myocardial infarction, heart murmur, valve prosthesis, or who take anticoagulant medication. There is some risk of infection of the tissue or bone surrounding the implant. A small number of implants fail every year, and some patients experience damage to nerves or other complications, depending on where the implants are placed in the jawbones.

The biggest contraindication is lack of available bone. This problem can usually be remedied utilizing various bone grafting techniques, as mentioned earlier. The procedure is recommended for those at least 16 years old, and there is no upper age limitation. Implants in the mandible, or lower jaw, enjoy a higher success ratio than those in the maxilla, or upper jaw, where bone may be softer. Dr. Weber, writing in the *Harvard Health Letter*, referred to one large study in which more than 4,500 implants were placed in the totally toothless jaws of 700 people. The five- to 15-year survival rate of the implant screws was 78 to 92 percent for those in the maxilla, as compared with 86 to 99 percent for implants placed in the mandible.[5]

Preparing for an implant. The most important preparation you can make if you are considering this process, is to select a qualified implant surgeon (an oral surgeon or periodontist) who has placed more than 200 implants and an experienced restorative dentist, or prosthodontist, who has fully and clearly planned the final tooth replacement in advance of the first surgical appointment. An inexperienced practitioner can produce an aesthetic nightmare that can be difficult if not impossible to correct.

Financial considerations. Currently, most dental plans do not cover the implant procedure. The usual reason given by the plans is that the procedure is still too new. Many dentists believe that this will change over time. Public confidence in the procedure justifiably continues to grow, and awareness continues to spread regarding the benefits. Meanwhile, prices range greatly according to case, geography, availability of specialists in a particular market, and qualifications of the practitioner. In New York City, a single tooth implant (crown and surgery) can cost over $5,000, whereas the replacement of all teeth in an upper or lower jaw can cost in excess of $35,000.

As more and more surgeons utilize this procedure, the rate of success continues to rise for dental implants. A quasi-experimental practice only a generation ago, today implant surgery successfully improves the comfort, nutrition, and self-esteem of over half a million Americans each year.

The dental implant has become dentistry's "miracle" procedure, and has proven conclusively that we can offer patients a second chance at the perfect smile.

THINGS TO REMEMBER

- Losing teeth can have both physiological and emotional consequences, but if you've lost teeth, there are a number of options available to you.

- Removable dentures are a solution that many people opt for, but not everyone adjusts to them well. It is also important to note that removable dentures need to be periodically relined by a dentist.

- Fixed prostheses or permanent bridges allow for a more comfortable lifestyle: You can eat or talk without worrying that they'll move. Bridgework is not for everyone, however, because it requires that the neighboring teeth be healthy.

- Dental implants are artificially created roots into which new artificial porcelain teeth can be screwed or cemented. They improve the self-esteem, comfort, and smiles of a growing number of Americans each year, but can be very expensive.

Chapter 5

A Brighter Smile

What You Can Do for Yourself

Much of this book focuses on how your dentist can help you obtain the smile you've always wanted. This chapter is all about what you can do for yourself. For all the advances made in recent years by restorative and cosmetic dentistry, the perfect smile really begins with you.

If you're among the many people who think that oral health means brushing your teeth twice a day, read on. This chapter is written with you in mind. You'll pick up some useful pointers on how to make your teeth look their best and improve your quality of life at the same time.

Most people think of brushing their teeth—if they think about it at all—as a dull chore; a routine learned in early childhood. Even though most people brush incorrectly, they don't want to spend time contemplating its nuances and subtleties.

Perhaps dentists bear some of the blame for that—some practitioners scold people more often than they should. If you're a dentist, and you're not mindful, the world becomes a parade of people with bad gums who sit in your chair and need to be reminded, one by one, to brush and floss after every meal.

A Word from the Doctor

When I began telling people I was writing a book called *The Perfect Smile*, they mostly responded with curiosity. I explained that the book would include a brief overview of how dentistry has advanced, and in particular, how new and constantly-evolving technologies are delivering Hollywood-caliber smiles—even to people who have been embarrassed by their smile all their lives.

Not smiling, when a smile is called for, can detract from how others see us. The absence of a smile often is interpreted as a hostile gesture, even if unintended. That said, people seemed interested in the book's concept, and would smile supportively and sometimes ask some questions.

When I came to the part about how it's the responsibility of each individual to maintain good dental habits, all bets were off. I watched as eyes glazed over. Heads continued to nod at appropriate intervals, but it was clear they had tuned out. Before long they would change the subject.

"Forget about it," an old friend told me. "You can't make a chapter on brushing your teeth interesting to anyone except maybe other dentists. And I'm not even sure about them."
Let's see whether we can change all that!

Of course, nobody wants to be scolded. So we've tried to make this chapter as painless as possible. There is probably nothing more important in this book than the information that follows—but only if you put it to use.

If you take good care of your teeth and gums, your chances of developing cavities and losing teeth are greatly reduced. Dr. Harold Loe, former director of the National Institute for Dental and Craniofacial Research of the National Institutes of Health said, "People think tooth loss is an inevitable part of aging. That is simply not true. All the diseases responsible for tooth loss are preventable."

Causes of Tooth Decay

In early childhood you were probably told to stay away from sugar because, it "causes tooth decay." This is true—the less processed sugar in your diet, the better.

The sugar found in most prepared foods—not just sweets—helps bacteria ferment. Fermenting bacteria generates byproducts called enzymes that cause the breakdown of soft tissue (such as your gums), the connective tissue beneath the surface, and hard tissue (such as the enamel on teeth and the bone that supports all your teeth). When this happens, it initiates a process referred to generally as "periodontal disease." (Several stages of periodontal disease are discussed later.)

Sugar combines with acids present in your mouth and helps bacteria form colonies that corrode tooth enamel. The main damage is done by a bacterium known as *S. mutans,* which converts sugar into sticky strands that cling to tooth surfaces and support colonies of bacteria. Like all living things, bacteria produce waste products. If these waste products are allowed to

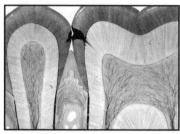
Tooth decay

remain in place, they bulk up and produce an acidic mass that's called plaque. The resulting acid build-up corrodes the surface of your teeth. This corrosion is what dentists call caries, and almost everyone else calls, simply, cavities. (It's safe to assume that if you ever hear anyone use the word *caries* in conversation, the speaker is a dentist.)

The word *cavity* inevitably makes people cringe. Years ago, a smart toothpaste company realized that they didn't have to go into a long, technical explanation to convince consumers to buy their brand. All they had to do was show a delighted youngster telling his mother the good news.

"Hey Mom! No cavities!"

What a wonderful thing to proclaim! But it isn't only a question of the brand of toothpaste you use. A twice-daily regimen of tooth-brushing *and* flossing, when done properly, removes the bacteria and food particles from your teeth.

Brushing and Flossing Go Hand in Hand

Brushing and flossing are both essential to achieving the perfect smile. Yet a surprising number of people who conscientiously brush twice a day find ways to put off flossing. Let me say it clearly here: If you don't floss, you are going to lose your teeth. It's that simple. Remember the old dental adage: "Floss between only those teeth you wish to keep."

Flossing regularly and carefully, as well as brushing properly, helps get rid of the 400 species of bacteria that live and ferment in the human mouth. If not tended to, these bacteria

THE HIDDEN CONNECTION

Heart Disease and Dental Plaque

Could the plaque that builds up on your gums cause a heart attack? A growing body of research suggests the answer could be yes.

In recent years, evidence has shown that heart disease—the leading cause of death in the United States—may originate in the mouth. For more than a decade, studies have suggested a correlation between plaque buildup in the mouth and such diseases as arteriosclerosis, or hardening of the arteries; stroke; and heart attack. Recent research also suggests that good dental hygiene can help prevent heart disease.

Doctors and other health experts have long associated heart disease with other factors, including smoking, lack of exercise, and excessive fat intake. Now, some have begun adding poor dental health to that list. A growing body of research demonstrates that plaque build-up can, under certain conditions, lead to heart disease. In 1989, a study done in Finland showed that patients being treated for myocardial infarctions had substantially more oral infections than did the patients in the control group.

In 1993, a study done in this country involving close to 10,000 adults indicated that periodontitis is a risk factor for developing coronary heart disease. Younger men were particularly at risk. In the study, men under 50 who had periodontal disease were nearly twice as likely to develop coronary heart disease as were their healthy-gummed peers. Another study completed that year showed that individuals who had lost teeth were more prone to develop heart disease than were people who held onto their original pearly whites.

Summarizing the results of a 1993 case-control study that examined dental health and heart conditions, Dr. Armind Grau concluded that people with dental problems were more than two and a half times as likely to suffer a stroke than were people who had maintained good dental health.

There is not yet consensus in the medical world regarding the connection between heart disease and gum disease. But there is enough evidence that if you need another reason to take better care of your teeth and gums, now you've got it.

gradually infect the gums and underlying bones, and eventually lead to both tooth loosening and tooth loss.

Did you know that the majority of Americans over 60 have lost most or all their teeth? It's true.

The presence of plaque on the gums and surface of the teeth can cause inflammation of the gums, commonly referred to as gingivitis (the medical term for gums is *gingiva*). Bacteria and their accumulated waste products have a toxic impact on the gum's soft tissue. Eventually the gums become red, swollen, irritated and prone to bleeding. Another sign of gingivitis is gums receding from the teeth, leaving sensitive root surfaces exposed.

If gingivitis goes untreated, inflammation spreads to the membranes around the base of the teeth, a condition known as periodontitis. Eventually, periodontitis can cause erosion of the bone in the jaw, resulting in tooth loss.

Careful and frequent brushing and flossing can prevent all of this. Surprisingly, most people don't know how to brush and floss properly. Let's start with the basics.

Toothpaste

The brands you'll find at the local supermarket or drugstore are all regulated by the Food and Drug Administration (FDA), and are proven to fight tooth decay when used properly. Most, but not all, have fluoride; it's a good idea to choose a brand with fluoride. For more on fluoride and fluoridation, see page 58.)

Toothbrush

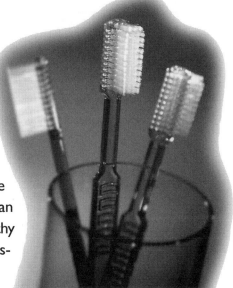

Toothbrushes are generally sold according to three levels of bristle stiffness: "hard," "medium," and "soft." Everyone has his or her own preferences, but we recommend choosing the "soft" brush and replacing it every two months or so. Soft bristles do the best job. Hard toothbrush bristles can cause damaging abrasion of healthy gum tissue, expediting gum "recession" via toothbrush abrasion.

Photo © Henry Schein, Inc.

A Word from the Doctor

An electric toothbrush can help you brush your teeth more effectively. There are many different models available: Some have circular heads of rotating bristles, while others have individual tufts of rotating bristles. Some models even have ultrasonic vibrating heads. They all work well.

What's great about the electric models is that all you have to do is hold the brush head on the tooth surface—the brush does the rest for you. The bristles move at a rate of 100 to 200 cycles a minute (depending on the brand you have); a speed that would be impossible to achieve with a manual toothbrush. Today, products such as the Crest SpinBrush make electric toothbrushes inexpensive enough for everyone to own and use one!

Brushing: A How-To Guide

Brushing right does not just mean brushing after meals. How we brush is every bit as important as when we brush, and dentists have found that most of us do not brush correctly or for long enough. You should brush for at least two minutes, concentrating on the inner surfaces of the teeth as well as parts that are visible when you smile. Here's how.

Squirt some fluoridated toothpaste on the bristles of your brush. Hold the brush so that the bristles face your teeth, and rotate your wrist so the bristles extend at a 45-degree angle.

Press the bristles against the gum line and press firmly—they should reach into the space between your teeth and gums. Brush back and forth ten times, firmly. Brush all teeth and gum lines in the lower jaw up and down ten times, and do the same for the insides of the teeth and gums. Repeat for the upper jaw. Then brush the chewing surfaces of the teeth.

Brush only as hard as it takes to get between your teeth. Brushing too hard can wear away gum tissue, and give you significant problems in later years.

Next, brush your tongue, extending the brush as far back into your mouth as you comfortably can. Stick your tongue out so the back is accessible. Brush up and down a few times. You might feel a gag reflex; after a few times doing this, you should lose that reflex. Don't forget to rinse your mouth after brushing your tongue.

Flossing: A How-To Guide

Flossing, though often neglected, should be an essential element of your oral health routine. Although flossing is not fun, it becomes less unpleasant if you use disposable plastic flossing units (they look a little like miniature slingshots) sold in many supermarkets and drug store chains. These little instruments get between teeth pretty well and make flossing easier, especially in the back of the mouth. If these instruments are uncomfortable, use the traditional line-wrapped-around-two-fingers method.

It's important to slide the floss all the way to gum level. Using an "up-and-down" motion, massage your gums, pressing the floss into the crevice between your teeth. Don't use a sawing motion, which can cause cuts in the gum tissue or grooves or ridges in the tooth or root surfaces.

When you floss, press firmly; a light touch doesn't do the job. There may be some bleeding if you floss sporadically. If bleeding continues, see your dentist; there may be a gum problem. Throw out the flossing stick, and use a new unit for the other jaw.

Some people cannot find the disposable flossing units in their store, or prefer to stick with the type of nylon flossing line they've used for years. If that's your preference, cut about 14 inches of floss and wrap it around the middle or index finger of each hand. Pull the floss tight using your thumb, keeping an inch or less taut between your fingers. Insert your fingers into your mouth and proceed as above, letting out new line as you move between teeth.

Mouthwash

If your dentist detects substantial decay between regular visits, he or she can recommend over-the-counter fluoride rinses or a prescription strength fluoride rinse, toothpaste and/or gel. Gel can be used on your normal toothbrush, or in some severe cases, it can be used in conjunction with fluoride trays that are worn for five minutes prior to retiring at night. Your dentist will recommend the method most appropriate for you.

Fluoride and Fluoridation

Fluoridation is a term that almost everyone has heard but few understand. Fluoridation is neither the elixir for perfect teeth nor the bogeyman some individuals have suggested it to be.

Fluorine is a natural compound whose ions have the effect of fortifying tooth enamel—fluoridation is the process of adding fluorine to another substance, commonly drinking water, toothpaste, or another dental care product. This fortification not only helps teeth resist decay, but also helps the calcium and phosphate in saliva replace minerals in the tooth enamel that have been lost to decay. This process is a major reason why Americans today suffer from dental decay less than past generations. More than half of the nation's school children are free of decay in their permanent teeth.

Moreover, fluoride used orally actually interferes with bacteria's ability to ferment and produce the toxins discussed earlier (See Causes of Tooth Decay on page 51). That's a marvelous benefit.

In its natural state, fluorine is a gas that combines with other elements to create a compound found in rocks and soil. As water rushes over rocks and soil it is fluoridated naturally, but sometimes inadequately for human needs. To make sure that our drinking water is amply fluoridated, most municipal water systems today add fluorine to the water supply. According to the U.S. Surgeon General, about two-thirds of the population drinks water that has been fluoridated.

Since the 1930s, multiple studies have shown that the public health benefits from drinking fluoridated water. Public health professionals agree that the evidence is incontestable. However, there continues to be political pressure exerted by some groups that believe the choice to fluoridate water should be made individually, rather than by government entities. Some groups suggest that public health is in fact threatened by fluoridation. But is it true?

Excess fluoride intake, while rare, can be toxic. More commonly, the result of excess fluoride ingestion is limited to vomiting, diarrhea, and irritation to the eyes. Children under the age of six who ingest excessive fluoride—theoretically, this might happen were a child to swallow a large amount of fluoridated toothpaste—are vulnerable to fluorosis, a condition in which the tooth's enamel is weakened, and the surface appears stained or speckled.

Fluoride is classified as a drug, and accordingly the Food and Drug Administration regulates its use. For this reason, products containing fluoride must note this fact clearly on all packaging.

These are real concerns to using fluoride. However, the consensus among dental and public health professionals is that the benefits outweigh the risks. While adverse effects of fluoridation are possible, the growing use of fluoride in much of our drinking water, and in the products sold on drug store and supermarket shelves, has provided an extraordinary benefit to the American mouth. The incidence of cavities has decreased enormously from past generations.

THINGS TO REMEMBER

- Cosmetic dentistry has made significant advances in recent years, but good oral hygiene is the first step to a brighter smile. Brushing and flossing one's teeth at least twice-a-day is essential.

- Remember that toothbrush bristles wear out and can cause more harm than good when they fray. Discard your old brush and purchase a new one every five to seven weeks for maximum cleaning and less gum abrasion.

- Make sure you brush your teeth correctly and for a long enough time. Don't forget to brush your gums and tongue.

- In addition to the traditional spool of floss, many other devices are now available to help you get between teeth.

- The growing use of fluoride in drinking water, toothpastes, and other products has improved America's oral health substantially in recent years, greatly reducing the occurrence of cavities.

Chapter 6

Eat Better, Smile Brighter

What's Sugar Got to Do with It?

As you're probably well aware, sugary foods are more likely to cause or speed up tooth decay than vegetables. If you can cut down on your sugar intake, you'll be doing yourself a favor—and not only in terms of dental health.

Unfortunately, eliminating processed sugar from your diet is easier said than done. Sugar consumption generally produces a sudden rush of energy and high spirits, a feeling often called a "sugar high." The feeling is addictive, and consequently, many of us have intense sugar cravings at one time or other. Many people subconsciously turn to sweets when they are feeling sad or unmotivated, knowing that after eating something sweet they'll feel better.

Now is a good time to evaluate the role of excess sugar consumption in your life. If you're diabetic and already follow a sugar-free diet, you can skip this section. If not, you might want to consider adapting such a diet, even if you don't suffer from a medical condition. People who reduce their sugar intake report better overall mental and physical health.

The Biology of Taste

Our taste buds can detect five flavors: sweet, sour, salty, bitter, and umami—the savory flavor of substances found in protein-rich foods. In America, the craving for sweets has traditionally been satisfied mainly by fresh fruit. For generations, a diet containing apples, oranges, bananas, and other glucose-laden fresh fruits was enough to satisfy the sweet tooth. Food created primarily from sugar was an occasional treat, usually reserved for the wealthy.

The American diet is no longer based on home-cooked meals. Today we often eat on the run and rely on others to prepare our food for us. The food industry adds ever-increasing amounts of processed sugar to foods and beverages that are bottled, canned, boxed, and shrink-wrapped for our consumption. Consequently, we expect nearly everything we eat to taste sweet—or at least sweeter than it tastes naturally.

Before reducing your sugar intake you must first examine the role that sweets play in your diet. If you feel excess sugar consumption is a problem for you, begin by tracking your sugar intake—you'll be surprised at how much sugar you actually eat every day. Many people conscientiously avoid the temptation to buy snacks in volume, and this is a good place to start. Do they ever eat donuts, or ice cream? Certainly, but only occasionally as a special treat. This reward based system doesn't work for everyone. If you're likely to indulge too many times a day, try keeping track of what, when, and why you snack in a notebook.

Once you begin to monitor your diet, you may see a pattern emerging. Most people find that their craving for sweets arises more or less on schedule. (The British expression. "I'm feeling eleven o'clockish," conveys the late-morning craving for something with jam on it. So it isn't just Americans!)

Snacking is often triggered by psychological need. Sugar gives us a high, and we crave it when we feel emotionally drained. If you suffer a setback, or someone behaves rudely to you, indulging in a candy bar makes you feel better—if only for a moment.

Beware of "Healthy" Sweets

Many sweets marketed as "healthy" are not actually good for you. Those "gummy" candies and "sour peaches" are highly cariogenic—they promote tooth decay and cause cavities.

Similarly, many so-called "fruit" juices are little more than sugar saturated beverages.

Many people find that breaking the sugar habit starts by realizing that temptation is temporary. If you can avoid giving in at the moment the craving occurs, fifteen or twenty minutes later the craving will pass. If that describes your behavior, keep a non-sweet snack food—like an apple—handy so you can have something to chew on when you feel a craving coming on.

There are a number of ways to combat sugar dependency and improve overall health. You might consider joining a gym or health club. Often people find that as they begin a conscientious exercise program, they find themselves craving sweets less often and less intensely. They start eating better as they begin to feel better about the shape they're in. They are less vulnerable to the need for that "sugar high."

Finally, if you're going to snack, brush and floss afterwards, just like after a meal.

Food That's Good for Your Teeth

No particular food has been shown to prevent tooth decay or gum disease. The belief that certain foods act as detergents, cleaning your teeth while you chew, is false. However, several vitamins and minerals associated with bone and tissue development can enhance dental health.

Calcium. This mineral is vital for tooth development and the maintenance of healthy bones—a strong jaw bone is essential for a healthy smile.

The average adult requires 1,200 milligrams of calcium daily, equivalent to two cups of skim milk, two cups of leafy vegetables, and a bowl of fortified cereal. Though calcium is often associated with milk, other good sources of calcium include fruit juices, nuts, tofu, and soy milk.

Vitamins. Vitamin C and vitamin B, including niacin, riboflavin, biotin and folate, are associated with building up resistance to gum disease, mouth sores, and oral inflammations. There is evidence that vitamin C can help promote healthy gums. Both vitamins are found in many fruits, vegetables, nuts and whole grain products, as well as in lean meat and dairy products.

Research suggests that vitamin E—found in beans, nuts, and whole grain foods—serves as an anti-gingivitis agent. Potassium, found in bananas, is also considered good for gums and teeth, as is vitamin D.

Fiber. High-fiber foods—including mangoes, celery, and winter squashes—give your mouth a kind of natural flossing. However they are not a substitute for actual flossing, as they leave fibers behind.

Supplements. Some preliminary studies indicate that supplements like coenzyme Q10 also help maintain healthy soft tissue, including the tissue in your gums. As part of the periodontal evaluation and treatment in our office, we encourage all patients, particularly those who have a propensity for bleeding gums or gum disease, to take a multivitamin, some food supplements like coenzyme Q10, and, of course, to not smoke.

In general, a healthy, well-balanced diet will help you in your efforts to achieve the perfect smile.

THINGS TO REMEMBER

- Keep track of your sugar intake. If you're among those who consume too much candy, try keeping a piece of fresh fruit nearby for moments when you crave something sweet.

- If you have a snack, remember to brush and floss afterward, just as you would after a meal.

- There are no foods that prevent tooth decay or gingivitis. However, calcium promotes tooth development and bone health, and vitamins B, C, D, and E have been shown to improve the health of your gums, and build your resistance to gum disease.

Chapter 7

Bad Breath

What Your Best Friend Won't Tell You

Halitosis. Bad breath. Do you have it? If you do, will anyone tell you?

Halitosis is the clinical name for a condition that afflicts about 80 million people worldwide. It's not the same as "morning breath"; it's not how your breath smells after you've eaten pepperoni pizza or a sauerkraut-laden hot dog.

One of the unfortunate realities of halitosis is that it develops gradually, so, you may be the last one to know you have the problem.

Bad breath is no joke. If you're afflicted with this problem, you may have detected the undesirable effect it has on other people. In social situations, you engage others in conversation only to discover that they invariably spot acquaintances over your shoulder, and suddenly find they need to rush away.

People with halitosis find that it affects their business as well. If people don't want to be near you, it's tough to get them to hire you, promote you, or buy your products. Not surprisingly, those with bad breath are more likely to suffer from depression than the general population.

A Word from the Doctor

Not long ago, I found out just how difficult it is for most people to tell someone close to them that they have bad breath. From time to time I take out advertising space in local publications to let people unfamiliar with our practice learn about the services we offer. Recently, I promoted a new and effective anti-halitosis program in our office. Since those with halitosis often don't know they have it, the ad was directed at people who share close quarters with them.

That single advertisement prompted more calls than any other ad we've ever run.

Unfortunately, many people with halitosis believe advertisements that promote mouthwashing solutions as an answer to their problems. These products offer a remedy by masking the odor in medicinal smells, rather than eliminating it.

Mouthwash products do not cure bad breath. In fact, sometimes they make it worse. Many contain alcohol, which dries out the mouth—dehydration worsens bad breath by restricting the flow of oxygen.

What Causes Bad Breath?

Bad breath is caused by food particles that get stuck in hard-to-reach places in the mouth. These particles can stick to the surfaces of teeth, between teeth, in pockets of gum surrounding teeth, on the tongue, or in oral appliances like dentures, braces, or crowns. The particles attract bacteria, which form colonies and begin to ferment. The fermentation produces volatile sulphur compounds—byproducts which have a distinct and unpleasant smell. People with bad breath show a high percentage of gasses like hydrogen sulfide or sulfur dioxide present in the carbon dioxide they exhale.

In many cases, bad breath is caused by inadequate oral hygiene. If you don't brush, floss, and scrape your tongue regularly, you may find yourself with offensive breath.

Taking Care of Your Tongue

Many people who are otherwise diligent about their oral hygiene somehow overlook the tongue, which is a potential breeding ground for fermenting bacteria. If you don't scrape your tongue regularly, bacteria may begin feasting on small particles of food caught between the papillae—natural fibers covering the tongue. In some cases of severe halitosis black spots are visible on the tongue where bacteria have set in. To offset this, ask your dentist for a high-quality tongue scraper, and use it regularly.

For many people, however, the problem isn't so simple. They brush. They floss. They scrape. Between meals. Before bed. After waking up. Yet their breath still undesirable. Why?

You can improve your bad breath by drinking more water and cutting back on coffee and smoking tobacco. Drinking eight glasses of water a day is recommended for general good health, and can help alleviate dry mouth—a condition that promotes bad breath by allowing odors to linger.

In some atypical cases, the problem is digestive—the acids in the stomach do not adequately break down foods such as onions, garlic, and pepper, or spicy condiments like curry or peppercorn. Dairy products can also be a problem, as can beans, especially when cooked without having been soaked in water to allow gas discharge. Making some of these dietary adjustments may help alleviate your digestive problems.

What's the Answer?

Studies have shown that classic bad breath does not originate in the digestive system. Halitosis, generally speaking, is a chronic issue that fails to respond to improvements in hygiene or dietary change. Then what can be done? Your dentist can be a source of help. Let's examine some of the available options.

Anti-halitosis products. In recent years a number of new products have become available to dentists, although most have not yet been made available for sale over the counter. These products use oxygenating agents such as chlorine dioxide, or neutralizing additives like zinc gluconate, to neutralize the sulphur compounds. These agents bond with the sulphur to produce an odor free gas, eliminating the problem.

Peroxide gels. In extreme cases, your dentist may recommend the use of a low concentration peroxide gel in a process similar to the one used in bleaching teeth. The peroxide oxygenates (in other words, pumps oxygen to) the deep crevices between your teeth. In this way, it cleanses the papillae on your tongue. This treatment has a very high rate of success, even for persistent halitosis. Please note that this is not a suggestion to rinse with straight or diluted peroxide from the pharmacy, which can cause many medical problems.

More visits with your dental hygienist. If the reactions of other people tell you that you have bad breath, I suggest you call your dentist today and schedule an appointment to have your teeth cleaned. A trained hygienist is able to reach and clean areas of your mouth that are difficult, if not impossible, for you to reach by yourself. The hygienist will also observe if food-trapping appliances or restorations (fillings, crowns, bridges) in your mouth need to be fixed, adjusted, or replaced. Performed three or four times a year, this service will go a long way in eliminating halitosis for many people and prevent it from recurring.

See a medical specialist. If halitosis persists, ask your dentist for a referral to an otolaryngologist—an ear, nose, and throat specialist (ENT). Many common medications used to treat everything from high blood pressure to depression produce mouth dehydration as a side effect, resulting in the formation of odorous gases. Mucous from postnasal drip contains dense proteins that are full of sulfur. A specialist will provide a thorough examination and medication review and should be able to identify the problem.

The bottom line? Halitosis is a problem that can be remedied. Bad breath need not be a deterrent in your pursuit of the perfect smile.

THINGS TO REMEMBER

- Over 80 million people worldwide suffer from halitosis, otherwise known as bad breath.

- Products such as mouthwash do not cure bad breath. Many contain alcohol, which dries the mouth and restricts the flow of oxygen, actually causing bad breath.

- Bad breath is caused by food particles that get stuck in hard-to-reach areas of the mouth.

- Food particles that get caught on papilae (natural fibers on your tongue) promote bacterial growth, which causes bad breath. Don't forget to brush and scrape your tongue after meals.

- If you have bad breath cut back on smoking or coffee consumption. Drinking water can also help freshen breath by alleviating dry mouth, which can allow odors to linger.

- A number of new products are now available to help neutralize the sulfur compounds that cause bad breath. Ask your dentist to recommend one.

- If you suffer from bad breath, try scheduling more visits with your dental hygienist. A trained hygienist is able to clean inside areas of the mouth that can be difficult to reach by yourself.

- If your halitosis does not improve, your dentist may refer you to an otolaryngologist—an ear, nose, and throat specialist—who can help identify the problem.

Maintaining Oral Health

Recognizing and Treating Problems, including TMJ

In many ways, your smile is a barometer of your overall health. After all, your body is a macro-system of interconnecting micro-systems. The bones, tissues, nerves, and blood vessels in your mouth connect with your entire body.

A number of medical conditions first manifest themselves in your mouth. Some are visible to you, while others require the intervention of a health care professional. In some cases your dentist is that professional, while in others you'll need a referral to a specialist.

In this chapter, we take a look at some syndromes and diseases that go beyond the teeth and gums, but may involve them as well.

Temporomandibular Joint Disorder (TMJ)

Temporomandibular Joint Disorder (TMJ or TMD) is associated with stress and involves pain that originates in the jaw or facial muscle. The temporomandibular joint, or TMJ, is the hinge between the skull and the jaw, the joint that opens and closes the mouth, making it possible for you to chew your food, swallow, speak, or laugh. "True" TMJ can manifest as the breakdown or deterioration of the cartilage in the disc that comprises the joint, or bony changes in the joint space or lower jawbone. Frequently, the condition mimics arthritis and may in fact involve arthritis. One early symptom can be jaw-popping, in which opening the mouth, as in a yawn, produces a clicking or popping sound.

"For years, I suffered with undiagnosed TMJ. My symptoms included tired, tense, and aching facial muscles (particularly around the jaw) and recurring pain that radiated from in front of my left ear, down my neck and through my shoulder. One day, as I was chewing, I felt a sharp popping in my jaw and the pain immediately became much worse. I saw Dr. Doundoulakis, who diagnosed TMJ and made a nightguard and a smaller appliance for me to wear. The results were startling: Within a few days of using these appliances, my symptoms had all but vanished."—M.A., New York City

Although we don't often realize it, the temporomandibular joint is one of the most important in the body, required for speaking, gesturing, and chewing. If the joint is injured by incessant tooth grinding, for example, it may respond favorably to anti-inflammatory drugs and arthritis medications, but surgery is recommended in advanced cases.

The disorder can result in complaints about difficulty chewing, talking, maintaining balance, hearing, headaches, and neck or back pain. In search of relief, Americans consult a wide range of practitioners, including chiropractors, nutritionists, pain specialists, and psychologists, as well as dentists, orthodontists, and maxillofacial surgeons (surgeons who specialize in the facial bones).

There is much difference of opinion about treatment options among these practitioners. Patients often consult one practitioner after another in search of relief, without satisfaction. The syndrome is often misdiagnosed and unsuccessfully treated. In some cases, orofacial pain can be treated with a combination of heat application, isometric exercises, muscle-relaxing medications, and stress reduction.

The surgical replacement of the joint is complex and should be considered only in the most extreme cases. Today, oral surgeons frequently utilize arthroscopic techniques, which can alleviate a patient's discomfort. This less invasive operation involves flushing out bone and tissue fragments with a saline solution and can substantially relieve discomfort in about 80 percent of cases, eliminating the need for replacement surgery. The syndrome has received much media attention lately, and is often over diagnosed. In fact, there is rampant disagreement among health care professionals about simply defining TMJ, let alone treating it effectively.

Is it caused by stress? Diet? Muscle problems? Poor posture? Hormones have even been implicated by some medical observers, in part because women of child-bearing age seem to constitute the largest single afflicted group.

"About 40 percent of Americans have some form of TMD, but only 5 to 10 percent have a problem that warrants treatment," Dr. James Fricton, co-director of the TMD and Orofacial Pain Division at the University of Minnesota, told *American Health* magazine[6].

Myofacial Pain Dysfunction (MFPD)

Nine of 10 patients who complain of TMJ may in fact be suffering from myofacial pain dysfunction (MFPD). MFPD is often a function of stress, subconscious muscle movement, and ill-positioned teeth.

Improving Occlusion

A patient with poor occlusion—a bite in which the upper jaw doesn't align properly with the lower jaw—may compensate for the problem by making nonnatural jaw movements. This can stretch the muscle beyond its limits and cause substantial muscle ache over time.

Poor occlusion can occur when a lost tooth isn't replaced and other teeth shift in the mouth to fill the void. Poor occlusion can also result if your teeth grew in misaligned or shifted at some point in adolescence or adulthood.

If you find yourself suffering from facial muscle pain, see your dentist. You might want to consider repositioning or reshaping your teeth to improve occlusion, and, of course, improve the overall aesthetic appearance of your mouth. A bite appliance or "night guard" can be fabricated to help teeth move freely and release tension in the facial muscles. An orthodontist can reposition your teeth, and a prosthodontist can reshape them.

Many adults react to the mention of orthodontics with a dismissive comment along the lines of, "No way, I'm not wearing braces for the next 18 months. I'm not in junior high school. I'll look silly."

New technologies have made braces a less visible—more palatable—alternative. One company has created a series of clear plastic orthodontic appliances that use digital imagery to guide the teeth through small, incremental changes in position.

Cosmetic rehabilitation is another alternative, which we discussed in detail in Chapter 2. A prosthodontist can also help you improve both your bite and your appearance quickly by reshaping and rebuilding your teeth, without using braces.

Tooth Grinding (Bruxism)

Tooth grinding, or bruxism, is a function of stress that often becomes a subconscious habit during sleep. Most people who grind their teeth are often unaware of the problem until the resultant pain becomes impossible to ignore. Symptoms are similar to those caused by TMJ. If ignored, bruxism can result in substantial muscle pain and increased difficulty eating and speaking.

Bruxism is a surprisingly common ailment, especially among people who live high-pressure lives—and more and more that includes most of us. Fortunately, the remedy is simple and relatively inexpensive: a mouth guard, or "night guard" as they are sometimes called. A customized mouth guard can cost anywhere from $250 to more than $500, depending on where you live and your dentist's fee structure. The mouth guard, which most people can wear without disturbing their sleep, protects teeth from wearing down even if the patient continues to grind. The mouth guard actually reduces these grinding movements by opening the bite a few millimeters, which adjusts muscle play and makes it more difficult to grind the jaws. Though devices like mouth guards can help alleviate the problem, they rarely stop it altogether.

Oral Cancer

Dentists are your first line of defense against oral cancer. Oral cancer screenings are performed during routine visits, although patients may not be aware of this. The dentist or hygienist examines three areas where oral cancer most commonly develops: the side of the tongue, the floor of the mouth, and the back of the upper hard or soft palate.

Oral cancer, especially of the malignant variety, occurs most commonly in patients who are regular smokers and heavy drinkers. If you have either one of these habits your likelihood of getting oral cancer increases considerably. If you have both these habits, your risk of getting oral cancer is 10 times greater than if you have either habit alone.

Diabetes

According to the American Diabetes Association, approximately 17 million people in the United States (6.2 percent of the population) have diabetes. The untreated diabetic patient will often have severe periodontal disease, because diabetes affects soft tissue. Exaggerated response to plaque (there may be spontaneous bleeding that is difficult to stop) is common, even when patients are diligent in their oral hygiene. For diabetic patients, routine dental visits are extremely important.

Whatever your age and medical history, your dental health demands that you receive appropriate dental care from a professional and that you participate in this on a daily basis by taking measures to keep your mouth healthy. Brush and floss after every meal and see your dentist on a regular basis. Don't be afraid to ask a lot of questions, or feel vain for deciding to change the look of your bite. Above all, it is important to realize that your dental health affects the appearance of your teeth and gums, and begins with the routine you follow and the choices you make. Eat, brush and floss with care and you'll be well on your way to a healthy perfect smile.

THINGS TO REMEMBER

- Some diseases first manifest themselves in your mouth, but may go beyond the teeth and gums.

- Temporomandibular disorder (TMD or TMJ) and Myofacial Pain Dysfunction (MFPD) are similar syndromes that involve pain in the jaw or facial muscles.

- TMD can cause jawbone cartilage to deteriorate, producing symptoms that often mimic arthritis. TMD is often treated with a combination of heat application, isometric exercises, muscle-relaxing medications, anti-inflammatory drugs, and stress reduction. In extreme cases, surgery may be necessary.

- Nine out of 10 patients who complain of TMD are actually suffering from MFPD, which is often a function of stress, subconscious muscle movement, and sometimes ill-positioned teeth.

- Poor occlusion—a bite in which the upper a lower jaws are misaligned—can cause severe muscle aches over time.

- If you suffer from orofacial pain you might consider repositioning or reshaping your teeth to improve occlusion.

- Bruxism, or tooth grinding, can mirror the symptoms of TMD, resulting in muscle pain and difficulty in eating and speaking. A night guard will often alleviate this problem.

- Regular smokers and heavy drinkers are more likely to develop oral cancer.

- People with diabetes often have periodontal disease. Because diabetes affects soft tissue, it is important that diabetics visit the dentist on a regular basis.

Appendix 1

Your dentist will outline several of the following dental implant treatment options, if you are missing one tooth, several teeth, or all your teeth. Before we review these options, let's look at the terminology the dentist will use in explaining his dental implant work.

An implant restoration consists of three stages. The first stage is the implant itself, which is placed in the bone by the surgeon and becomes osseointegrated. Once osseointegration has occurred, there must be a mechanism to extend the implant through the soft tissues. This extension that goes through the gum tissue (or second stage) is called an abutment. Abutments come in a variety of different types and shapes, each designed to manage the particular clinical situation. The third stage, or restoration, is based on the use of an implant part called the gold cylinder. The gold cylinder becomes incorporated into the final crown or bridge and provides the base or seat for the implant crown. The final crown or fixed bridge is then either cemented to a custom post or retained by a small screw.

Types of Implant Restorations

Single Tooth Replacement or Crown
The single tooth replacement is one of the most challenging esthetic restorations. Today it is the most common procedure for replacing one missing tooth.

Indications

Conservation of tooth structure.
A common alternative to single tooth replacement is the conventional tooth bridge, connecting a "fake" tooth to adjacent teeth. This requires the removal of tooth structure and

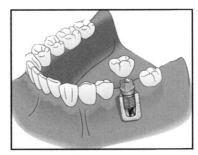

Single tooth replacement

possible root canal treatment. Placement of a single implant avoids the preparation or cutting of an additional tooth, and avoids root canal.

Contraindications

Restoration of adjacent teeth is necessary. If adjacent teeth require extensive rehabilitation, a fixed bridge should be considered.

Poor supporting bone. As with any implant, adequate bone must be available.

Small Span Bridge

Indication

Several teeth are missing in the front or back of the mouth and adjacent teeth are unprepared or virgin natural teeth. When some or all the teeth are missing, this is known as edentulism. Small span, fixed bridges eliminate the need for removable partial dentures and provide stable abutments for fixed

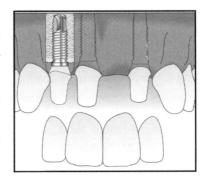

Small span bridge

bridgework. This includes bridges solely supported by implants or by a combination of implants and the natural teeth connected by some type of retrievable mechanism (not as popular anymore).

Contraindication
Poor supporting bone. As with any implant, adequate bone must be available.

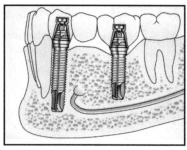

Full fixed bridge

Full Arch Fixed Bridge (Entire Jaw)

Full arch fixed bridge type prostheses can be constructed on osseointegrated implants, provided there is adequate supporting structure and that an acceptable esthetic result can be realized. Under ideal circumstances, a patient can convert from a complete removable denture to a totally fixed bridge, enjoying the use of non-removable teeth.

Indications
Adequate ridge height. Full arch crown and bridge type restorations can only be considered for totally edentulous patients when there is adequate ridge height to produce a normally sized and shaped final crown. Minimal resorption (melting away of bone) of the bony ridge permits the final restoration to be tooth-like in size and shape.

Contraindications
Moderate to severe ridge resorption. When there has been moderate to severe bone loss or resorption, a fixed

restoration requires replacement of more than just tooth crowns. Root dimension and bone height must be replaced as well. This is difficult to achieve using a conventional crown and bridge type restoration because of framework considerations.

The need for extensive cantilevering (adding posterior teeth that are suspended by the bridge). In totally edentulous patients, implants are generally placed in the front of the lower jaw and the upper sinus. This requires extensive cantilevering to provide some posterior bite. To avoid these long extensions, a bone graft in the sinus may be indicated.

Inadequate lip support. The prosthesis may not adequately support the lip, resulting in a soft tissue crease under the nose. (see *overdenture type*)

Hybrid Prosthesis

The osseointegrated hybrid prosthesis involves components of both the complete removable denture and the traditional fixed bridge. It consists of a metal framework supporting denture teeth. Denture acrylic is processed around the denture teeth, connecting them to the metal framework. This allows replacement for the lost bone and gum tissue as well as root structures in the patient with moderate to severe bone loss (resorption). Generally, these restorations are associated with extensive cantilevering in the back areas of the bridge. It is commonly referred to as the "Classic

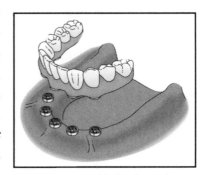

Osseointegrated hybrid prosthesis

Branemark" design, named after the pioneering orthopedic surgeon who discovered the process of osseointegration.

Indications

Totally edentulous arches with moderate to severe resorption. The hybrid prosthesis is used in moderately to severely resorbed edentulous patients because it provides maximum flexibility when positioning the teeth, despite the location of the implants. The denture teeth can be placed in the proper position to provide lip support and occlusal function; this position may not be directly over the implants themselves.

Cantilever and shock absorption requirements. Acrylic occlusion provides some shock absorption, which is particularly necessary in extensive cantilevers (10 to 15 millimeters) situations.

Used mostly in lower jaws where all teeth are missing. In some special cases, can also be used in upper jaws when all teeth are missing.

Contraindications

Minimal ridge resorption. When there is minimal ridge resorption, the hybrid prosthesis is contraindicated because the open surface beneath the hybrid prosthesis will be displayed during function.

Potential occurence of speech problems when the hybrid prosthesis is used in the upper jaw.

Overdenture Prosthesis

The denture type of implant restoration is a cost-effective method that provides the best lip support and speech control. Denture implant restorations are generally constructed by connecting the implant abutments with a gingival bar and using an overdenture clip for retention.

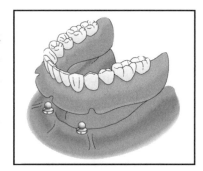

Overdenture Prosthesis

Indications

Lip support requirements. Especially in the upper arch, a fixed prosthesis may be inadequate to provide sufficient lip support in the anterior regions because of resorption of the bony ridges. The use of an overdenture provides the option of extending the pink plastic flange to properly support the lip. This will maximize esthetics and facial contours.

Patient concerns. Patients who have worn removable dentures for many years sometimes feel that such devices allow for more effective cleansing of the mouth. These patients feel more comfortable having a removable prosthesis and are primarily concerned about prosthesis stability.

Financial concerns. The overdenture is usually a less expensive alternative for the replacement of multiple osseointegrated implants in an edentulous arch (where all the teeth are missing). Because the bar requires fewer laboratory procedures, the cost is considerably reduced.

Contraindications

Patient concerns. Many patients have a psychologic aversion to wearing a removable device. This aversion can be extremely strong and these patients may try to avoid removable prostheses at all costs.

Hyperactive gag reflexes. The overdenture sometimes requires extension onto the palate area of the upper jaw and tongue areas of the lower jaw. Placement into these areas may activate the patient's gag reflexes.

Poor supporting bone. As with any implant, adequate bone must be available.

Appendix 2
Resources

Web Sites

www.cosmeticdentalny.com
Award-winning Web site of Dr. James H. Doundoulakis, DMD, MS, FACD. This site provides information on the art of cosmetic dentistry, prosthodontics, tooth whitening, and implant options. It also lists the office location, telephone numbers and policies of his practice.

www.cosmetic--dentist.com
Cosmetic Dentist Directory provides the quickest, most efficient method of finding a qualified dentist who emphasizes dental aesthetics and dental restorations.

www.dental--implants.com
A directory of dental restoration, reconstruction and implant dentistry professionals, including prosthodontists, implant periodontists, and oral and maxillofacial surgeons.

www.dentistry.com
A privately operated organization that provides information-based resources, catering to dental professionals and consumers. Consumers receive access to the largest search engine of dental professionals and products, as well as opportunities to contact featured Dentistry.com specialists through an online consultation page.

Organizations

Academy of General Dentistry
211 East Chicago Avenue, Suite 900
Chicago, IL 60611-1999
Phone: (312) 440-4300
www.agd.org
The Academy of General Dentistry strives to represent the interests of general dentists and improve the quality of comprehensive dental services, health promotion and wellness. The Academy's Web site offers resources on oral health topics, an opportunity to post oral health related questions, and a Find a Dentist directory.

Academy of Osseointegration
85 West Algonquin Road, Suite 550
Arlington Heights, IL 60005-4425
Phone: (800) 656-7736
Fax: (847) 439-1919
www.osseo.org
The Academy of Osseointegration is an international dental implant organization with over 4,200 members. The Academy is interested in bringing together individuals of different backgrounds to share experience and knowledge regarding implants to advance the field of osseointegrated implants.

American Academy of Cosmetic Dentistry

5401 World Dairy Drive

Madison, WI 53718

Phone: (800) 543-9220

www.aacd.com

The AACD provides literature as a service to consumers, so that you may learn more about cosmetic dentistry.

American Academy of Esthetic Dentistry

401 North Michigan Avenue

Chicago, IL 60611

Phone: (312) 321-5121

www.estheticacademy.org

The AAED is comprised of distinguished individuals from virtually every facet of the dental profession. Members are educators who share a common interest in esthetics and excellence in the quality of patient care.

American Academy of Pediatric Dentistry

211 East Chicago Avenue, Suite 700

Chicago, IL 60611-2663

Phone: (312) 337-2619

Fax: (312) 337-6329

www.aapd.org

The AAPD is an organization with 5,600 members representing the specialty of pediatric dentistry. Pediatric dentists are specialists dedicated to the oral health of children and patients with special health care needs. The AAPD Web site offers information to parents and a Find a Pediatric Dentist directory.

American Academy of Periodontology
737 North Michigan Ave., Suite 800
Chicago, IL 60611-2690
Phone: (312) 787-5518
www.perio.org
The American Academy of Periodontology (AAP) is a 7,800-member association of dental professionals specializing in the prevention, diagnosis and treatment of diseases affecting the gums and supporting structures of the teeth and in the placement and maintenance of dental implants.

American Association of Oral and Maxillofacial Surgeons
9700 West Bryn Mawr Avenue
Rosemont, IL 60018-5701
Phone: (847) 678-6200
www.aaoms.org
The American Association of Oral and Maxillofacial Surgeons (AAOMS), is a not-for-profit professional association serving the professional and public needs of the specialty of oral and maxillofacial surgery.

While oral and maxillofacial surgeons are best known for extracting wisdom teeth, they also reconstruct faces shattered by trauma, surgically correct misaligned jaws, and perform cancer surgery of the face and neck.

American College of Prosthodontists

211 East Chicago Avenue, Suite 1000

Chicago, IL 60611

Phone: (312) 573-1260

Fax: (312) 573-1257

www.prosthodontics.org

Founded in 1970, ACP is a non-profit educational and scientific organization for the specialty of prosthodontics.

The ACP Web site provides consumers with information about prosthodontics and a Find a Prosthodontist directory.

American Dental Association (ADA)

211 East Chicago Avenue

Chicago, IL 60611-2678

Phone: (312) 440-2500

Fax: (312) 440-7494

www.ada.org

The ADA is the professional association of dentists committed to the public's oral health, ethics, science and professional advancement; leading a unified profession through initiatives in advocacy, education, research and the development of standards.

The ADA Web site provides consumers with lists of oral health topics and ADA Seal products, as well as a Find a Dentist directory, tips for teachers, and children's games.

American Dental Hygenists' Association
444 North Michigan Avenue, Suite 3400
Chicago, IL 60611
Phone: (312) 440-8900
www.adha.org
ADHA is the largest professional organization representing the interests of dental hygienists. The ADHA Web site provides information on oral health, periodontal disease, bad breath, nutrition, tooth whitening and offers tips on proper brushing and flossing.

Centers for Disease Control and Prevention
1600 Clifton Road
Atlanta, GA 30333
Phone: (404) 639-3534
(800) 311-3435
www.cdc.gov
The Centers for Disease Control and Prevention (CDC) is the leading federal agency for protecting the health and safety of people. The CDC Web site provides a comprehensive resource library of oral health information that can be browsed by topic.

Food and Drug Administration (FDA)
5600 Fishers Lane
Rockville, Maryland 20857-0001
Phone: (888) INFO-FDA
www.fda.gov
The FDA is the federal agency responsible for ensuring that foods are safe, wholesome and sanitary; human and veterinary drugs, biological products, and medical devices are safe and effective; cosmetics are safe; and electronic products that emit radiation are safe. The FDA also ensures that these products are honestly, accurately and informatively represented to the public.

National Institute of Dental and Craniofacial Research
NIDCR Public Information and Liaison Branch
45 Center Drive, MSC 6400
Bethesda, MD 20892-6400
Phone: (301) 496-4261
www.nidcr.nih.gov
The mission of the National Institute of Dental and Craniofacial Research (NIDCR) is to promote the general health of the American people by improving their oral, dental and craniofacial health. The NIDCR Web site provides an index of oral health topics that includes information on fluoride, TMJ, gum disease, tooth decay, oral cancer, spit tobacco, orofacial pain, sealants, and more.

Appendix 3
Glossary

A

abutment An implant component delivered to the patient at the time the final implant crown is being placed. Available in various sizes, lengths, shapes and materials (mostly metal or aluminum oxide crystal).

ADA American Dental Association, the leading voice and credentialing body of the profession and discipline of dentistry in the United States.

alloy Mixture of silver and mercury called amalgam that has been used for over seventy years, the most routine dental restorations worldwide.

amalgam Better known as silver fillings. Amalgam is an alloy of silver, tin, and mercury. See **alloy.** The most common filling material used today.

artificial root A dental implant. Substitute for the natural tooth root.

B

bonding Tooth-colored fillings made from a resin called composite. Used to fill small cavities or chips, or to reshape teeth. See **composite.** The bonding process is the technique in which composite resin is attached or placed onto or in the tooth.

Branemark Professor Per Ingvar Branemark is a Swedish orthopedic surgeon who discovered the process of osseointegration. He is generally referred to as the father of modern implant dentistry.

bruxism Habitual tooth grinding, usually occurring during sleep. Stress related.

C

calculus Commonly known as tartar. Calculus are the mineralized colonies of bacteria and their by-products, all of which are destructive to teeth and gum tissue.

carbamide/peroxide The most commonly used ingredient for home tooth bleaching.

caries Destruction of teeth caused by bacteria. Dental decay.

cavity See **caries.** The generic term for dental decay.

composite Composite resin is a white filling material, more commonly known as bonding. These white fillings not only better resemble teeth, but they also do not contain mercury as silver fillings do.

cosmetic dentistry Branch of dentistry devoted to the artistic and scientific enhancement of a person's smile and oral health.

crown A prosthetic that restores the anatomy, function, and esthetics of a natural tooth.

D

dental implant An artificial device placed within the bone that provides support for artificial teeth. Artificial substitute for the natural tooth root. See **artificial root.**

dental phobia An exaggerated, conditioned and/or illogical fear of dental treatment.

dentures A partial or complete set of artificial teeth. Removable dentures must come out for cleansing at bedtime and after meals. Usually made of strengthened acrylic resin.

Duchenne smile A genuine smile that utilizes the *zygomaticus* muscle in the cheek. Named after the pioneering French neurologist whose work led to an understanding of the physiology of the smile.

E

endodontist A specialist trained to handle difficult root canal treatment.

endosseous implant See **dental implant.**

F

fixed bridges Also known as permanent bridges. Function like natural teeth, because they are not removable. Are attached to the adjacent teeth on either side of the missing tooth.

fluoridation Process of adding fluorine to another substance, commonly drinking water, toothpaste, or other dental care products. Helps teeth resist decay.

fluorine Natural compound whose ions have the effect of fortifying tooth enamel.

G

gingivectomy A gingivectomy, or gum lift, is a procedure in which the dentist removes excess gum tissue.

gingivitis Inflammation of the gums. One of the first signs of periodontal disease. At this stage, bone loss has not yet begun, and is reversible.

H

halitosis Clinical condition of bad breath.

hygienist Dental professional auxiliary who performs professional cleanings, prophylaxis, and other similar procedures in the dental office, under the supervision of a dentist.

L

laminates A very thin porcelain veneer or wafer that covers only the front surface and edge of the tooth, protecting it and improving its appearance.

M

mandible Lower jawbone.

myofacial pain dysfunction (MFPD) A disorder that involves pain in the facial muscles. MFPD is often a function of stress, subconscious muscle movement, or ill-positioned teeth.

N

novocaine Term most commonly used for dental anesthetic. In actuality, dentists do not use novocaine anymore, due to its high risk for allergic reaction. More commonly, dentists are using other types of anesthetics, such as lidocaine or mepivicaine.

O

occlusion The relation between the surfaces of your teeth when in contact, also known as your 'bite.'

oral surgeon A specialist who removes impacted teeth, performs various jaw surgeries, and surgically places dental implants.

orbicularis oculi The muscle that surrounds the eye. When you grin, you work both the *zygomaticus* and *orbicularis muscles*.

orthodontist A specialist trained to straighten multiple teeth, utilizing braces or other devices.

osseointegration Bonding between the dental implant and the jawbone.

P

permanent bridges *See* **fixed bridges.**

periodontist A specialist trained to treat advanced gum and periodontal disease, perform gum surgery, and surgically place dental implants.

periodontitis Inflammation and irreversible disease in the membranes around the bone and base of the teeth. Results when gingivitis goes untreated. At this stage there is bone loss around the teeth.

plasma arc light The most effective light source used today for non-laser power tooth whitening in the dental office. The most recognized dental centers advertising tooth whitening utilize a PAC light.

post A device that is often necessary following root canal therapy to help strengthen the remaining tooth tissue, prior to the placement of a crown.

prophylaxis The routine professional dental cleaning includes prophy, or thorough removal of plaque from between and around all the teeth.

prosthodontist A specialist trained to provide the restoration, beautification, and/or replacement of teeth.

restoration Any prosthetic device that restores or replaces lost teeth, tooth structure, or tissue.

ridge modification Procedure in which bone or bone substitute is grafted onto the jaw to prepare for implant placement.

risorius smile A smile that appears false and calculated, named after the facial muscle that is used to pull the lips back but not up.

root canal A therapeutic process of removing diseased tissue to save a tooth. Root canal therapy removes diseased nerve tissue in the root of a tooth and allows the patient to continue normal use and function pain free.

S

scaling Scaling (and root planning) is done to remove plaque and calculus from around and beneath the gum line. In some cases, it must be performed with dental anesthetic.

silver fillings *See* **alloys.**

sinus augmentation or sinus lift Procedure in which bone is grafted within the maxillary sinus to prepare for implant placement.

specialty One of the ADA recognized dental specialities in dentistry, including dental radiology, endodontics, maxillofacial and oral surgery, oral pathology, orthodontics, pedodontics, periodontics, and prosthodontics. Cosmetic and implant dentistry are not recognized ADA specialities.

streptococcus mutans Bacterium that converts sugar into sticky strands that cling to tooth surfaces. A major cause of dental decay or caries.

T

tartar *See* **calculus.**

temporomandibular joint Joint that opens and closes the mouth.

temporomandibular joint disorder (TMJ) A disorder that involves pain in the jaw joint or facial muscles. TMJ can cause jawbone cartilage to deteriorate, producing symptoms that often mimic arthritis.

titanium The most popular biocompatible material used in implant rehabilitation. Can be either commercially pure or used as an alloy.

tooth reshaping A procedure that involves scraping a wafer-thin slice of enamel from your tooth to remove uneven or chipped edges and other imperfections.

V

veneer A very thin sheet of porcelain made to cover the front surface and edge of the tooth, protecting it and preserving its appearance. *See* **laminates.**

Z

zygomaticus muscle The *zygomaticus* muscle connects the corners of the mouth with the cheekbone. It is the primary muscle involved in smiling.

Notes

[1] "The Perfect Smile: A Guide to Great-Looking Teeth," Wendy Korn, *Ladies Home Journal*, v102, October 1985.

[2] "Goodbye, Dentures: Improved Dental Implants Gaining Favor," Julie Bain, *The New York Times*, September 2001.

[3] A Tooth For A Tooth." Hans-Peter Weber, *Harvard Health Letter*, v18, n6, April, 1993.

[4] Ibid

[5] Ibid

[6] "Jaw Pain: How To Navigate the Treatment Minefield," *American Health* magazine, November 1993.

Special Thanks

The Authors and Publisher would like to thank the following organizations and companies for generously providing artwork and information for *The Perfect Smile*. We gratefully acknowledge their contributions.

3i Implant Innovations, Inc.
4555 Riverside Drive
Palm Beach Gardens, FL 33410
www.3i-online.com

American College of Dentists
839J Quince Orchard Boulevard
Gaithersburg, Maryland 20878-1614
www.facd.org

American Dental Association
Division of Communications
211 East Chicago Avenue
Chicago, IL 60611
www.ada.org

Crest Dental Products
The Proctor and Gamble Company
Cincinnati, OH 45202
www.dentalcare.com

Sullivan-Schein Dental
A Henry Schein Company
135 Duryea Road
Melville, NY 11747
www.henryschein.com

Nobel Biocare USA, Inc.
22715 Savi Ranch Parkway
Yorba Linda, CA 92887
www.nobelbiocareusa.com

Index

A

Abutment, 96
Academy of General Dentistry, 90
Academy of Osseointegration, 90
Alloy, 96
Alternative payment plans, 16
Amalgam fillings, 28, 96
American Academy of Cosmetic Dentistry, 91
American Academy of Esthetic Dentistry, 91
American Academy of Pediatric Dentistry, 91
American Academy of Periodontology, 92
American Association of Oral and Maxillofacial Surgeons, 92
American College of Prosthodontists, 93
American Dental Association, 93, 96
American Dental Hygienists' Association, 94
Appointment availability, 14
Appointment reliability, 15
Artificial root, 96
Artificial teeth, 42
Aural environment, providing a calm, 9

B

Bad breath, 68–73, 99
Biofeedback, use of, 9
Bleaching, tooth, 31–36
Bonding, 28–29, 96

D

E

F

G

Gingivectomy, 29–30, 99
Gingivitis, 54, 55, 99
Grinding, tooth, 78
Group practice, 18

H

Halitosis, 68–73, 99
Holistic approaches to dental care, 8–9
Hybrid prosthesis, 85–86
Hygienist, 99
Hypnosis, use of, 9

I

Implant restorations, 82–88
Implants, dental, 42–47, 98
Insurance plan coverage, 15–16

L

Laminates, 30–31, 99

M

Malocclusions, correcting, 36–37
Mandible, 99